The Bearded Dragon Bible

Definitive Handbook for Beginners: Expert Care and Ownership Tips for a Happy,
Healthy Bearded Dragon

Leo Herptor

1. Introduction to bearded dragons

Bearded dragons, scientifically known as Pogona, are fascinating reptiles that have captured the hearts of many pet enthusiasts around the world. Originating from the arid and semi-arid regions of Australia, these creatures have adapted remarkably well to a variety of environments, making them resilient and relatively easy to care for in captivity. The bearded dragon's name derives from the spiny scales that cover their throats, which can puff up and darken, resembling a beard, especially when they feel threatened or are engaging in social displays. This unique feature, along with their docile nature and manageable size, makes them a popular choice among reptile keepers.

The evolutionary journey of bearded dragons is a testament to their adaptability and resilience. Over millions of years, these reptiles have evolved to thrive in some of the harshest environments on Earth. Their ancestors were part of a diverse group of reptiles that roamed the ancient supercontinent of Gondwana. As the continents drifted apart, the ancestors of modern bearded dragons found themselves in Australia, where they continued to evolve, developing traits that allowed them to survive in the continent's diverse climates. This evolutionary history has endowed bearded dragons with a range of physical and behavioral adaptations that make them well-suited to life both in the wild and in captivity.

Anatomically, bearded dragons are equipped with several features that aid their survival. Their bodies are covered in rough, spiny scales that provide protection from predators and harsh environmental conditions. They have strong limbs and sharp claws that enable them to climb and dig, essential behaviors for finding food and creating burrows. Their long tails, which can be used for balance and communication, are another distinctive feature. Internally, bearded dragons have a highly efficient digestive system that allows them to extract maximum nutrients from their food, an adaptation to their often sparse and unpredictable natural diet.

Behaviorally, bearded dragons are known for their calm and inquisitive nature. They are diurnal, meaning they are active during the day and sleep at night, which aligns well with the daily routines of their human caretakers. In the wild, they are solitary creatures, coming together only to mate. However, in captivity, they can exhibit a range of social behaviors, including head bobbing, arm waving, and beard puffing, which are used to communicate with other dragons and their human companions. Understanding these behaviors is crucial for providing appropriate care and ensuring the well-being of these reptiles.

As pets, bearded dragons offer a unique blend of companionship and low-maintenance care. Unlike more traditional pets such as dogs or cats, bearded dragons do not require constant attention and can be left alone for longer periods, making them ideal for busy individuals or those who travel frequently. They are also relatively easy to handle and can form strong bonds with their owners, often recognizing and responding to their presence. This combination of traits makes them particularly appealing to first-time reptile owners and those looking for a pet that is both engaging and manageable.

Choosing your first bearded dragon is an exciting step, but it requires careful consideration. Prospective owners should look for healthy, active dragons with clear eyes, clean skin, and a good appetite. It is also important to consider the dragon's age and size, as younger dragons require more frequent feeding and monitoring, while older dragons may have established routines and behaviors. Additionally, understanding the specific needs of bearded dragons, such as their dietary requirements, habitat setup, and health maintenance, is essential for providing the best possible care.

In summary, bearded dragons are remarkable creatures with a rich evolutionary history and a range of unique physical and behavioral traits. Their adaptability and resilience have made them popular pets, offering a rewarding experience for those willing to invest the time and effort into understanding their needs. This introductory chapter sets the stage for a deeper exploration of bearded dragon care, providing the foundation for the detailed instructions and insights that follow in this comprehensive guide. Whether you are a first-time owner or an experienced reptile keeper, "The Bearded Dragon Bible" will equip you with the knowledge and confidence to ensure your bearded dragon thrives in your care.

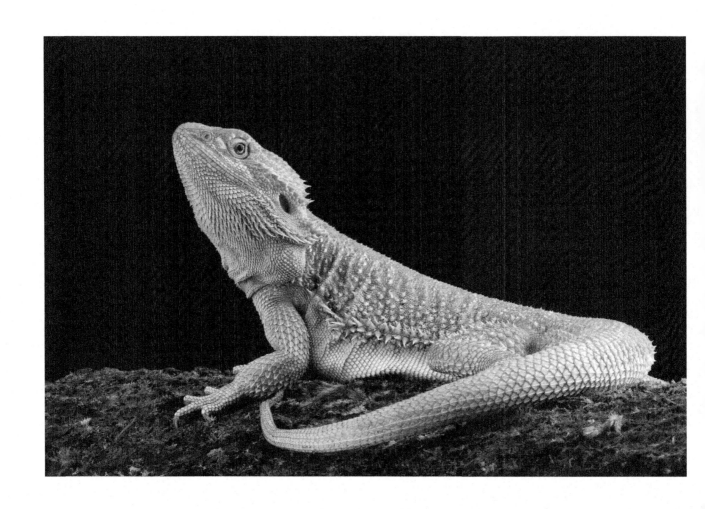

1.1 The origins of bearded dragons

Bearded dragons, scientifically known as Pogona, are fascinating reptiles that have captured the hearts of pet enthusiasts around the world. To truly appreciate these remarkable creatures, it is essential to delve into their origins, tracing their lineage back to the arid landscapes of Australia. The story of the bearded dragon begins millions of years ago, in the harsh and unforgiving deserts of the Australian continent. These regions, characterized by extreme temperatures, sparse vegetation, and limited water sources, provided the perfect backdrop for the evolution of a species uniquely adapted to survive in such an environment.

The bearded dragon's ancestors were part of a diverse group of reptiles that roamed the ancient supercontinent of Gondwana. As Gondwana began to break apart, the landmass that would eventually become Australia drifted northward, carrying with it a unique array of flora and fauna. Over millions of years, the bearded dragon's ancestors adapted to the changing climate and landscape, developing traits that would ensure their survival in the increasingly arid conditions.

One of the most significant adaptations of the bearded dragon is its ability to thermoregulate. In the scorching heat of the Australian desert, maintaining an optimal body temperature is crucial for survival. Bearded dragons have evolved to be ectothermic, meaning they rely on external sources of heat to regulate their body temperature. They bask in the sun to warm up and seek shade or burrow into the ground to cool down. This behavior is not just a survival mechanism but also a testament to their incredible adaptability.

The bearded dragon's distinctive appearance is another result of its evolutionary journey. Their rough, spiky skin serves as both camouflage and protection. The coloration of their scales, ranging from sandy browns to vibrant oranges, allows them to blend seamlessly into their desert surroundings, evading predators and ambushing prey. The "beard" for which they are named is a flap of skin under their throat that can be puffed out and darkened when they feel threatened or are trying to assert dominance. This display is not only a defense mechanism but also a form of communication within their species.

The diet of bearded dragons has also evolved to suit their environment. In the wild, they are opportunistic feeders, consuming a variety of insects, small vertebrates, and vegetation. This varied diet ensures they receive the necessary nutrients to thrive in a habitat where food sources can be scarce. Their ability to switch between carnivorous and herbivorous diets depending on availability is a remarkable adaptation that has contributed to their success as a species.

The bearded dragon's reproductive strategies are equally fascinating. In the wild, breeding typically occurs during the warmer months when conditions are most favorable for the survival of their offspring. Females lay clutches of eggs in burrows they dig in the sand, providing a safe and stable environment for incubation. The temperature of the nest plays a crucial role in determining the sex of the hatchlings, a phenomenon known as temperature-dependent sex determination. This adaptation ensures a balanced sex ratio within the population, contributing to the species' long-term viability.

The journey of the bearded dragon from the ancient deserts of Australia to becoming one of the most popular reptile pets in the world is a testament to their resilience and adaptability. Their ability to thrive in captivity is a direct result of their evolutionary history. Understanding their origins not only deepens our appreciation for these remarkable creatures but also informs how we care for them as pets. By replicating their natural habitat and providing a diet that mimics their wild counterparts, we can ensure that our bearded dragons live healthy and fulfilling lives.

In recent years, scientific research has provided valuable insights into the behavior and physiology of bearded dragons. Studies have shown that they possess a level of intelligence and social complexity that was previously underestimated. For example, research conducted by the University of Lincoln in the UK demonstrated that bearded dragons are capable of social learning, a trait more commonly associated with mammals and birds. In the study, bearded dragons were able to learn how to open a sliding door by observing a trained conspecific, highlighting their ability to learn from their peers.

Another fascinating aspect of bearded dragon behavior is their use of body language to communicate. In addition to their beard displays, they use a variety of gestures such as head bobbing, arm waving, and tail curling to convey different messages. These behaviors play a crucial role in social interactions, whether it be establishing dominance, signaling submission, or attracting a mate. Understanding these behaviors is essential for anyone looking to provide the best care for their bearded dragon, as it allows for better interpretation of their needs and emotions.

The conservation status of bearded dragons in the wild is another important consideration. While they are not currently listed as endangered, habitat destruction and climate change pose significant threats to their natural populations. Efforts to protect their habitats and ensure sustainable practices in the pet trade are crucial for the long-term survival of the species. By supporting conservation initiatives and promoting responsible pet ownership, we can contribute to the preservation of these incredible reptiles for future generations.

In conclusion, the origins of bearded dragons are a captivating tale of evolution and adaptation. From their ancient ancestors in Gondwana to their current status as beloved pets, bearded dragons have demonstrated remarkable resilience and versatility. By understanding their historical roots and the environmental challenges they have overcome, we can better appreciate the unique qualities that make them such extraordinary companions. Whether basking in the sun or displaying their impressive beards, bearded dragons continue to captivate and inspire those who have the privilege of sharing their lives with these remarkable reptiles.

1.2 Evolutionary journey

The evolutionary journey of the bearded dragon is a fascinating tale of adaptation and survival that spans millions of years, tracing back to the ancient landscapes of Australia. These remarkable reptiles, scientifically known as Pogona, have undergone significant evolutionary changes that have enabled them to thrive in diverse and often harsh environments. To truly appreciate the bearded dragon's current form and behavior, it is essential to understand the key adaptations and evolutionary milestones that have shaped their existence.

The origins of bearded dragons can be traced back to the late Cretaceous period, approximately 100 million years ago, when the supercontinent Gondwana began to break apart. This geological event led to the isolation of the Australian landmass, creating a unique environment for the evolution of its flora and fauna. Early ancestors of the bearded dragon were likely small, insectivorous reptiles that roamed the arid and semi-arid regions of ancient Australia. Fossil evidence suggests that these early reptiles possessed primitive features, such as elongated bodies and simple limb structures, which were well-suited for a life of burrowing and foraging.

As the Australian continent continued to drift and its climate became increasingly arid, the bearded dragon's ancestors faced new environmental challenges. The scarcity of water and the need to regulate body temperature in extreme heat drove the evolution of several key adaptations. One of the most significant adaptations was the development of a robust, spiny body covered in scales. These scales not only provided protection from predators but also played a crucial role in thermoregulation by reflecting sunlight and reducing water loss through the skin. The characteristic "beard" of the bearded dragon, a spiny throat pouch that can be inflated and darkened, likely evolved as a means of communication and defense. When threatened, a bearded dragon can puff up its beard, making itself appear larger and more intimidating to potential predators.

Another critical adaptation in the evolutionary journey of the bearded dragon is their highly efficient metabolic system. Bearded dragons are ectothermic, meaning they rely on external sources of heat to regulate their body temperature. This adaptation allows them to conserve energy and survive in environments with limited food resources. Their ability to enter a state of brumation, a form of hibernation, during periods of extreme cold or drought further enhances their survival prospects. During brumation, a bearded dragon's metabolic rate slows down significantly, allowing it to endure prolonged periods without food or water.

The bearded dragon's diet has also evolved to suit its environment. While early ancestors were primarily insectivorous, modern bearded dragons are omnivorous, consuming a varied diet that includes insects, small vertebrates, fruits, and vegetables. This dietary flexibility has allowed them to exploit a wide range of food sources, increasing their chances of survival in fluctuating environmental conditions. The evolution of strong, sharp claws and a powerful jaw has enabled bearded dragons to efficiently capture and consume their prey, while their keen sense of vision helps them detect movement from a distance.

Social behavior and communication have played a significant role in the evolutionary success of bearded dragons. These reptiles are known for their complex social interactions, which include head bobbing, arm waving, and color changes. These behaviors are used to establish dominance, attract mates, and communicate with other bearded dragons. The evolution of these intricate social behaviors has likely contributed to the bearded dragon's ability to form stable social groups and avoid conflicts, thereby enhancing their overall fitness and reproductive success.

Research into the genetic makeup of bearded dragons has provided further insights into their evolutionary history. Studies have revealed that bearded dragons possess a unique set of genes that regulate their development, behavior, and physiology. For example, the gene responsible for the development of their distinctive beard is linked to hormonal changes that occur during stress or mating. Understanding the genetic basis of these traits has not only deepened our knowledge of bearded dragon evolution but also provided valuable information for their conservation and care.

The evolutionary journey of the bearded dragon is a testament to the power of natural selection and adaptation. From their humble beginnings as small, insectivorous reptiles to their current status as one of the most popular exotic pets, bearded dragons have demonstrated remarkable resilience and versatility. Their ability to thrive in diverse environments, coupled with their unique physical and behavioral adaptations, has ensured their survival for millions of years. As we continue to study and care for these captivating creatures, we gain a deeper appreciation for the intricate processes that have shaped their evolution and the vital role they play in our understanding of the natural world.

In conclusion, the evolutionary journey of the bearded dragon is a rich and complex narrative that highlights the interplay between environmental pressures and adaptive responses. By examining the fossil record, genetic data, and behavioral studies, we can piece together the story of how these remarkable reptiles have evolved to become the resilient and adaptable creatures we know today. As bearded dragon owners and enthusiasts, it is our responsibility to honor this evolutionary legacy by providing the best possible care and ensuring their continued survival in both captivity and the wild.

1.3 Anatomy and physiology

Bearded dragons, scientifically known as Pogona, are fascinating reptiles that have captured the interest of pet enthusiasts worldwide. Their unique anatomy and physiology are key to understanding their behavior, care needs, and overall well-being. One of the most distinctive features of bearded dragons is their "beard," a spiky collar around their necks that can inflate and darken when the dragon feels threatened, stressed, or is trying to assert dominance. This beard is not just for show; it plays a crucial role in their social interactions and communication.

The bearded dragon's body is covered in rough, spiny scales that provide protection against predators in their natural habitat. These scales are not just a defensive mechanism; they also help with thermoregulation. Bearded dragons are ectothermic, meaning they rely on external heat sources to regulate their body temperature. Their scales can absorb and retain heat, which is vital for their metabolic processes. This is why providing a proper heat source in their enclosure is crucial for their health.

Their head is triangular with a broad, flat shape, which aids in their ability to burrow and hide from predators. The eyes are positioned on the sides of their head, giving them a wide field of vision. This placement allows them to be vigilant and aware of their surroundings, which is essential for both hunting and avoiding threats. Bearded dragons have excellent eyesight and can see in color, which helps them identify food and potential mates.

The mouth of a bearded dragon is equipped with sharp, small teeth that are perfect for their omnivorous diet. They have a sticky tongue that they use to catch insects, much like a chameleon. Their jaw muscles are strong, allowing them to crush hard-shelled insects and chew plant material effectively. Understanding their dental structure is important for providing the right types of food and ensuring they receive the necessary nutrients.

Bearded dragons have a robust and muscular body, with strong limbs that are adapted for climbing and digging. Their claws are sharp and curved, providing a good grip on various surfaces. This physical strength is not just for mobility; it also plays a role in their social behavior. During mating season, males will often engage in physical displays and combat to win over a female. These displays can include head bobbing, arm waving, and even physical wrestling.

The tail of a bearded dragon is another significant feature. It is long and muscular, aiding in balance and agility. The tail can also be used as a weapon against predators or rivals. In some cases, bearded dragons can lose their tail as a defense mechanism, although this is less common compared to other lizards. The tail also stores fat, which can be used as an energy reserve during times of scarcity.

Internally, bearded dragons have a unique respiratory system that allows them to thrive in arid environments. They have a series of air sacs that help them maximize oxygen intake and maintain hydration. Their lungs are highly efficient, allowing them to survive in conditions where water is scarce. This adaptation is crucial for their survival in the wild and must be considered when setting up their habitat in captivity.

The digestive system of a bearded dragon is adapted to process a varied diet of insects, vegetables, and fruits. They have a relatively short digestive tract, which means they need a diet that is easy to digest and rich in nutrients. Providing a balanced diet is essential for their health, as improper nutrition can lead to serious health issues such as metabolic bone disease.

Bearded dragons also have a well-developed nervous system, which is evident in their complex behaviors and interactions. They are highly intelligent reptiles capable of learning and adapting to their environment. This intelligence makes them fascinating pets, as they can recognize their owners and respond to various stimuli. Their brain structure is adapted for processing sensory information, which is crucial for their survival and social interactions.

Reproductive anatomy is another important aspect of bearded dragon physiology. Males have hemipenes, which are paired reproductive organs, while females have a single oviduct. Understanding their reproductive anatomy is essential for breeding and ensuring the health of both the male and female dragons. Breeding bearded dragons requires careful attention to their health, diet, and environmental conditions to ensure successful mating and healthy offspring.

In summary, the anatomy and physiology of bearded dragons are complex and fascinating, with each feature playing a crucial role in their survival and well-being. From their distinctive beard and spiny scales to their robust limbs and efficient respiratory system, every aspect of their physical structure is adapted to their environment and lifestyle. Understanding these features is essential for providing the best care and ensuring that your bearded dragon thrives in captivity. Whether you are a first-time owner or an experienced reptile enthusiast, appreciating the intricacies of bearded dragon anatomy will deepen your connection with these remarkable creatures and help you provide the best possible care.

1.4 Behavioral traits

Bearded dragons, with their endearing personalities and intriguing behaviors, have captivated the hearts of reptile enthusiasts worldwide. Understanding their unique behavioral traits is essential for any bearded dragon owner, as it provides insights into their well-being and helps foster a deeper bond between pet and owner. One of the most fascinating aspects of bearded dragon behavior is their method of communication, which includes a variety of physical gestures and postures. Head-bobbing, for instance, is a common behavior where a bearded dragon rapidly moves its head up and down. This action can signify different things depending on the context. In males, head-bobbing is often a display of dominance or a courtship behavior aimed at attracting females. Conversely, slow head-bobbing can indicate submission, particularly in younger or less dominant dragons. Understanding these nuances helps owners interpret their pet's social interactions and manage their environment accordingly.

Another notable behavior is arm-waving, where a bearded dragon raises one of its front legs and moves it in a circular motion. This gesture is typically a sign of submission or acknowledgment of another dragon's dominance. It is often observed in younger dragons or females in the presence of more dominant males. Arm-waving can also be a response to perceived threats, signaling that the dragon is not a threat and wishes to avoid confrontation. Observing and recognizing this behavior can help owners create a more harmonious environment, especially if they have multiple dragons.

Bearded dragons are also known for their sun-basking habits, which are crucial for their thermoregulation and overall health. In the wild, these reptiles spend a significant amount of time basking in the sun to absorb heat and UVB rays, which are essential for their metabolism and calcium absorption. In captivity, providing a basking spot with appropriate temperature and UVB lighting is vital to mimic their natural habitat. Owners may notice their dragons flattening their bodies and spreading their limbs to maximize surface area exposure to the heat source. This behavior, known as "pancaking," is an indication that the dragon is thermoregulating effectively.

Another intriguing behavior is glass-surfing, where a bearded dragon repeatedly runs along the sides of its enclosure, often appearing to try to climb the glass. This behavior can be a sign of stress, boredom, or an inadequate environment. It may indicate that the enclosure is too small, lacks sufficient hiding spots, or that the dragon is seeking more stimulation. Addressing these issues by providing a larger habitat, enriching the environment with decor and hides, and ensuring proper temperature gradients can help reduce glass-surfing behavior.

Bearded dragons also exhibit a range of feeding behaviors that can provide insights into their health and preferences. For example, a healthy dragon will actively hunt and chase live prey, displaying quick reflexes and keen eyesight. In contrast, a lack of interest in food or lethargic feeding behavior may indicate health issues or environmental stressors. Observing feeding habits can help owners detect early signs of illness and make necessary adjustments to diet or habitat conditions.

Brumation is another significant behavior observed in bearded dragons, akin to hibernation in mammals. During brumation, a dragon's activity levels decrease, and it may eat less or stop eating altogether. This period of dormancy typically occurs in response to seasonal changes in temperature and daylight hours. Understanding brumation is crucial for owners, as it requires adjustments in care routines, such as reducing feeding frequency and ensuring the dragon has a cool, dark place to rest. Recognizing the signs of brumation and differentiating them from illness is essential for maintaining the dragon's health during this natural process.

Social interactions with humans and other animals also play a significant role in bearded dragon behavior. These reptiles can form bonds with their owners and may exhibit behaviors that indicate trust and comfort, such as climbing onto their owner's hand, sitting calmly on their shoulder, or closing their eyes when being petted. Building this trust requires gentle handling, consistent routines, and positive reinforcement. Conversely, signs of stress or discomfort, such as puffing up their beard, hissing, or attempting to flee, indicate that the dragon needs more time to acclimate or that the handling approach needs to be adjusted.

In addition to these behaviors, bearded dragons have unique ways of expressing curiosity and exploration. They may tilt their heads to better observe their surroundings, investigate new objects with their tongues, or dig in the substrate to create burrows. Providing an enriched environment with opportunities for exploration, such as climbing branches, rocks, and varied textures, can stimulate these natural behaviors and contribute to the dragon's mental and physical well-being.

Understanding and interpreting these behavioral traits is essential for any bearded dragon owner. It not only enhances the care and management of these fascinating reptiles but also deepens the bond between pet and owner. By observing and responding to their dragon's behaviors, owners can create a supportive and enriching environment that promotes the health and happiness of their scaly companion. Whether it's recognizing the significance of head-bobbing, providing appropriate basking spots, or understanding the nuances of brumation, each aspect of bearded dragon behavior offers valuable insights into their needs and preferences. As owners become more attuned to these behaviors, they can ensure their bearded dragon thrives in captivity, leading to a rewarding and fulfilling pet ownership experience.

1.5 Bearded dragons as pets

Bearded dragons have become increasingly popular as pets, and for good reason. These fascinating reptiles, with their prehistoric appearance and gentle demeanor, offer a unique pet ownership experience that is both rewarding and manageable. One of the primary reasons bearded dragons are favored as pets is their docile nature. Unlike many other reptiles, bearded dragons are known for their calm and friendly disposition. They rarely exhibit aggressive behavior, making them suitable for handling and interaction, even for beginners. This trait is particularly appealing to pet owners who seek a companion that can be easily tamed and socialized.

In addition to their temperament, bearded dragons are of a manageable size, typically growing to about 18-24 inches in length. This size makes them easy to house and care for, as they do not require the extensive space that larger reptiles might need. Their relatively small size also makes them less intimidating to new reptile owners, who may be apprehensive about handling larger or more aggressive species. The ease of caring for bearded dragons is another significant factor contributing to their popularity. Unlike some exotic pets that have highly specialized and demanding care requirements, bearded dragons have relatively straightforward needs. They thrive in a well-maintained habitat that mimics their natural environment, with appropriate temperature gradients, UVB lighting, and a suitable substrate. Their diet is also relatively simple, consisting of a mix of insects, vegetables, and occasional fruits. This simplicity in care makes them an ideal choice for individuals who may not have extensive experience with reptiles but are eager to learn and provide proper care.

Case studies and research have shown that bearded dragons can form strong bonds with their owners. For example, a study conducted by the University of Lincoln found that bearded dragons can recognize their owners and exhibit behaviors that suggest a level of social interaction and recognition. This ability to bond with their human caretakers adds to their appeal, as owners can enjoy a sense of companionship and interaction that is often associated with more traditional pets like dogs and cats. Another reason bearded dragons are favored as pets is their relatively long lifespan. With proper care, bearded dragons can live for 10-15 years, providing a long-term companion for their owners. This longevity allows for a deeper bond to develop over time, as owners can watch their bearded dragon grow and thrive throughout different life stages.

The bearded dragon's unique appearance also contributes to their popularity. Their spiky beard, which they can puff out when threatened or excited, along with their distinctive scales and vibrant colors, make them visually striking pets. This exotic look appeals to individuals who are drawn to the unusual and the extraordinary, offering a pet that stands out from the more common household animals. Furthermore, bearded dragons are relatively low-maintenance compared to other exotic pets. They do not require constant attention or interaction, making them suitable for individuals with busy lifestyles. While they do need regular feeding, habitat maintenance, and occasional handling, they are generally content to bask in their enclosure and explore their surroundings at their own pace. This balance of independence and interaction makes them an attractive option for those who want a pet that fits into their schedule without demanding constant supervision.

In terms of health, bearded dragons are hardy reptiles that, with proper care, can avoid many common health issues. Regular veterinary check-ups, a balanced diet, and a well-maintained habitat can help prevent problems such as metabolic bone disease, respiratory infections, and parasites. This resilience adds to their appeal, as owners can feel confident in their ability to provide a healthy and happy life for their pet. The educational aspect of owning a bearded dragon is also a significant draw for many pet owners. Caring for a bearded dragon offers a unique opportunity to learn about reptile biology, behavior, and ecology. This educational experience can be particularly enriching for children and young adults, fostering a sense of responsibility and curiosity about the natural world. Many schools and educational programs have incorporated bearded dragons into their curriculum, using them as a hands-on learning tool to teach students about reptiles and their care.

Community and social interaction are also important factors in the popularity of bearded dragons as pets. There are numerous online forums, social media groups, and local clubs dedicated to bearded dragon enthusiasts. These communities provide a wealth of information, support, and camaraderie for new and experienced owners alike. Sharing experiences, tips, and stories with fellow bearded dragon owners can enhance the pet ownership experience and provide valuable insights into the best practices for care and enrichment. Additionally, bearded dragons are often featured in reptile expos and pet shows, where owners can connect with breeders, veterinarians, and other experts. These events offer opportunities to learn more about bearded dragon care, discover new products and technologies, and meet other enthusiasts who share a passion for these captivating reptiles.

In conclusion, bearded dragons are favored as pets for a multitude of reasons, including their docile nature, manageable size, ease of care, and unique appearance. Their ability to bond with their owners, relatively low maintenance requirements, and educational value further enhance their appeal. With a supportive community of fellow enthusiasts and a wealth of resources available, bearded dragon ownership can be a fulfilling and enriching experience. Whether you are a first-time reptile owner or an experienced enthusiast, bearded dragons offer a rewarding and engaging pet ownership journey that is both unique and accessible.

1.6 Choosing your first bearded dragon

Choosing your first bearded dragon is an exciting and crucial step in your journey as a reptile owner. This subchapter will guide you through the process, ensuring you make an informed decision that will lead to a happy and healthy relationship with your new scaly friend. When selecting your first bearded dragon, it's essential to identify healthy specimens. A healthy bearded dragon should have bright, clear eyes, a clean vent area, and smooth, unblemished skin. Their body should be well-proportioned, with no visible signs of injury or deformity. Observe their behavior; a healthy bearded dragon will be alert and active, showing curiosity about their surroundings. It's also important to check for any signs of respiratory issues, such as wheezing or mucus around the nose and mouth. Understanding the different morphs and colors of bearded dragons can also play a significant role in your selection process. Bearded dragons come in a variety of morphs, which are genetic variations that affect their color, pattern, and scale structure. Some popular morphs include the classic or wild type, which has a natural brown or tan coloration, and the leatherback, which has smoother scales. Other morphs, such as the hypomelanistic (hypo) and translucent (trans), exhibit reduced pigmentation and unique eye colors. Each morph has its own set of care requirements and potential health issues, so it's important to research and understand these differences before making a decision. Sourcing your bearded dragon from a reputable breeder is crucial to ensure you are getting a healthy and well-cared-for pet. Reputable breeders will provide detailed information about the dragon's lineage, health history, and care requirements. They will also be able to answer any questions you may have and offer ongoing support. Avoid purchasing bearded dragons from pet stores or online marketplaces where the animals may have been subjected to poor conditions or inadequate care. Instead, seek out breeders who are members of recognized reptile associations or who have positive reviews from other reptile enthusiasts. When visiting a breeder, take the time to observe the living conditions of the bearded dragons. The enclosures should be clean and well-maintained, with appropriate lighting, heating, and substrate. The dragons should have access to fresh water and a varied diet that includes both insects and vegetables. Ask the breeder about their feeding and care routines, and request to see any health records or documentation for the dragon you are interested in. It's also a good idea to ask for references from other customers who have purchased bearded dragons from the breeder. In addition to physical health, consider the temperament of the bearded dragon you are choosing. Bearded dragons are known for their docile and friendly nature, but individual personalities can vary. Spend some time handling and interacting with the dragon to gauge their comfort level with human interaction. A well-socialized bearded dragon will be more likely to adapt to their new environment and bond with you as their owner. Be patient and gentle during this process, as it may take some time for the dragon to become accustomed to being handled. Another factor to consider when choosing your first bearded dragon is their age. Juvenile bearded dragons are often more affordable and easier to find, but they require more intensive care and monitoring as they grow. Adult bearded dragons, on the other hand, may be more expensive but are generally hardier and have established eating and behavior patterns. If you are a beginner, starting with a juvenile bearded dragon can be a rewarding experience, as you will have the opportunity to watch them grow and develop. However, be prepared for the additional care and attention they will need during their early stages of life. It's also important to consider the long-term commitment of owning a bearded dragon. These reptiles can live for 10 to 15 years with proper care, so be sure you are ready for the responsibility of providing for their needs over the long term. This includes regular feeding, habitat maintenance, and veterinary care. Bearded dragons require a specific environment to thrive, including appropriate lighting, heating, and humidity levels. Make sure you are prepared to invest in the necessary equipment and supplies to create a suitable habitat for your new pet. In conclusion, choosing your first bearded dragon is a significant decision that requires careful consideration and research. By identifying healthy specimens, understanding different morphs and colors, sourcing from reputable breeders, and considering factors such as temperament, age, and long-term commitment, you can ensure a successful and rewarding experience as a bearded dragon owner. Remember, the key to a happy and healthy bearded dragon is providing them with the best possible care and environment, so take the time to educate yourself and make informed choices. With the right preparation and dedication, you will be well on your way to becoming a confident and knowledgeable bearded dragon owner.

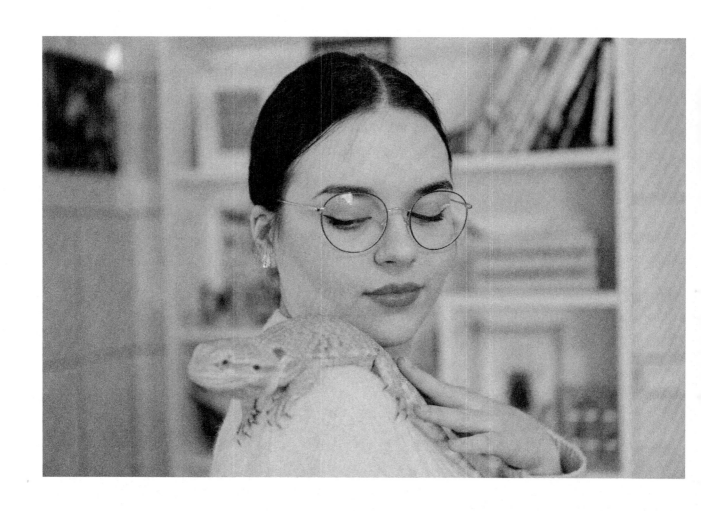

2. Setting up your bearded dragon's habitat

Setting up your bearded dragon's habitat is a crucial step in ensuring the health and happiness of your new scaly companion. A well-designed habitat mimics the natural environment of bearded dragons, which are native to the arid regions of Australia. This chapter will provide detailed guidance on creating the perfect living environment for your bearded dragon, covering everything from choosing the right tank to temperature control, lighting, and essential equipment.

The first step in setting up your bearded dragon's habitat is selecting the appropriate tank. Bearded dragons require ample space to move around, bask, and explore. A tank that is too small can lead to stress and health issues. For a juvenile bearded dragon, a 20-gallon tank may suffice, but as they grow, they will need a larger enclosure. An adult bearded dragon requires at least a 40-gallon tank, with a 75-gallon tank being ideal for optimal comfort. The tank should be made of glass or acrylic to provide clear visibility and easy cleaning. It should also have a secure, ventilated lid to prevent escapes and ensure proper airflow.

Once you have chosen the right tank, the next step is setting up the substrate. The substrate is the material that lines the bottom of the tank and serves as the flooring for your bearded dragon. There are several options for substrates, each with its pros and cons. Reptile carpet is a popular choice because it is easy to clean and reduces the risk of impaction, a condition where the dragon ingests substrate material and becomes unable to pass it. Other options include paper towels, newspaper, and ceramic tiles. Loose substrates like sand and wood chips should be avoided, especially for young dragons, as they pose a higher risk of impaction.

Temperature control is a critical aspect of your bearded dragon's habitat. Bearded dragons are ectothermic, meaning they rely on external heat sources to regulate their body temperature. The tank should have a temperature gradient, with a basking area on one side and a cooler area on the other. The basking area should be maintained at 95-110°F, while the cooler side should be around 75-85°F. At night, the temperature can drop to 65-75°F. To achieve this gradient, you will need a combination of heat lamps and ceramic heat emitters. Place a basking lamp above the basking area to create a hotspot, and use a thermometer to monitor the temperatures in different parts of the tank.

In addition to heat, bearded dragons require proper lighting to thrive. UVB lighting is essential for their health, as it helps them synthesize vitamin D3, which is necessary for calcium absorption. Without adequate UVB exposure, bearded dragons can develop metabolic bone disease, a serious and often fatal condition. A UVB bulb should be placed inside the tank, within 12-18 inches of the basking area, and should be replaced every six months, as its effectiveness diminishes over time. It is also important to provide a day-night cycle by turning off the lights at night to mimic natural conditions.

Installing hides and decor in the tank is another important aspect of creating a comfortable habitat for your bearded dragon. Hides provide a sense of security and a place for your dragon to retreat when it feels stressed or needs to cool down. You should have at least two hides in the tank, one in the basking area and one in the cooler area. Additionally, adding branches, rocks, and other decor items can create a stimulating environment and encourage natural behaviors like climbing and basking. Make sure that all decor items are securely placed to prevent them from falling and injuring your dragon.

Ongoing maintenance and cleaning of the habitat are essential to keep your bearded dragon healthy. Spot clean the tank daily by removing uneaten food, feces, and shed skin. Perform a thorough cleaning of the tank and all its contents at least once a month. This involves removing your dragon from the tank, disinfecting all surfaces with a reptile-safe cleaner, and rinsing everything thoroughly before returning your dragon to its home. Regular maintenance helps prevent the buildup of harmful bacteria and parasites.

In conclusion, setting up your bearded dragon's habitat requires careful planning and attention to detail. By choosing the right tank, setting up the appropriate substrate, maintaining proper temperature and lighting, and providing hides and decor, you can create a safe and comfortable environment for your bearded dragon to thrive. Regular maintenance and cleaning are also crucial to ensure the long-term health and well-being of your pet. With the right setup, your bearded dragon will have a happy and healthy life, bringing you joy and companionship for years to come.

2.1 Choosing the right tank

When embarking on the journey of bearded dragon ownership, one of the most critical decisions you'll make is choosing the right tank. This choice will significantly impact your pet's health, well-being, and overall happiness. Bearded dragons, known for their docile nature and captivating behaviors, require a habitat that not only meets their physical needs but also provides an environment that mimics their natural surroundings. The importance of selecting an appropriate tank cannot be overstated, as it lays the foundation for all aspects of your bearded dragon's care.

First and foremost, let's discuss the size of the tank. Bearded dragons are active reptiles that require ample space to move, explore, and engage in natural behaviors. A common mistake among new owners is opting for a tank that is too small, which can lead to a host of health issues and behavioral problems. For a baby bearded dragon, a 20-gallon tank may suffice temporarily, but as they grow, they will need significantly more space. Adult bearded dragons, which can reach lengths of up to 24 inches, should be housed in a tank that is at least 75 gallons. However, many experts recommend going even larger, with a 120-gallon tank being ideal. This extra space allows for a more dynamic and enriching environment, giving your bearded dragon room to roam, bask, and hide.

When considering tank types, there are several options available, each with its own set of advantages and disadvantages. Glass tanks are a popular choice due to their visibility and ease of cleaning. They provide a clear view of your bearded dragon, allowing you to monitor their behavior and health closely. However, glass tanks can be heavy and may not retain heat as efficiently as other materials. On the other hand, wooden vivariums with glass fronts offer better insulation, helping to maintain the necessary temperature gradients within the tank. These vivariums can be customized with various finishes and designs, making them an attractive addition to your home decor. Another option is PVC or plastic enclosures, which are lightweight, durable, and excellent at retaining heat. These tanks are often used by professional breeders and serious hobbyists due to their practicality and ease of maintenance.

Ventilation is another crucial factor to consider when choosing a tank. Bearded dragons require a well-ventilated environment to prevent the buildup of humidity and ensure a steady supply of fresh air. Tanks with mesh tops or built-in ventilation systems are ideal, as they allow for proper airflow while still maintaining the necessary temperature and humidity levels. It's important to strike a balance between ventilation and heat retention, as bearded dragons thrive in a warm, dry environment.

In addition to size and material, the tank's layout and design play a significant role in your bearded dragon's overall well-being. A well-designed tank should include a variety of features that cater to their natural behaviors and needs. For instance, bearded dragons are ectothermic, meaning they rely on external heat sources to regulate their body temperature. Therefore, the tank should have a designated basking area with a heat lamp or ceramic heat emitter to provide the necessary warmth. This basking spot should be positioned at one end of the tank, creating a temperature gradient that allows your bearded dragon to move between warmer and cooler areas as needed.

Furthermore, bearded dragons are known for their love of climbing and exploring. Including branches, rocks, and other climbing structures in the tank can help stimulate their natural instincts and provide mental and physical enrichment. These elements not only make the tank more visually appealing but also encourage exercise and prevent boredom. Additionally, providing multiple hiding spots is essential for your bearded dragon's sense of security. Hides can be created using commercially available reptile hides, cork bark, or even DIY options like small cardboard boxes. These hiding spots allow your bearded dragon to retreat and feel safe, reducing stress and promoting overall health.

Lighting is another critical aspect of tank setup. Bearded dragons require both UVB and UVA lighting to thrive. UVB lighting is essential for the synthesis of vitamin D3, which in turn aids in calcium absorption and prevents metabolic bone disease. UVA lighting, on the other hand, helps regulate their behavior and appetite. It's important to choose high-quality UVB bulbs and replace them every six months, as their effectiveness diminishes over time. The lighting should be positioned to cover the entire length of the tank, ensuring that your bearded dragon receives adequate exposure throughout the day.

Substrate selection is another important consideration when setting up your bearded dragon's tank. The substrate is the material that lines the bottom of the tank and can significantly impact your pet's health. There are various substrate options available, each with its own set of pros and cons. Loose substrates like sand and gravel are often discouraged due to the risk of impaction if ingested. Instead, opt for safer alternatives like reptile carpet, paper towels, or tile. These substrates are easy to clean and reduce the risk of impaction, making them a safer choice for your bearded dragon.

In conclusion, choosing the right tank for your bearded dragon is a multifaceted decision that requires careful consideration of size, material, ventilation, layout, lighting, and substrate. By providing a spacious, well-designed, and properly equipped tank, you can create a thriving environment that meets your bearded dragon's physical and behavioral needs. This investment in their habitat will pay off in the form of a healthy, happy, and active pet, allowing you to enjoy the unique companionship and fascinating behaviors of your bearded dragon for years to come.

2.2 Setting up the substrate

When it comes to setting up the substrate for your bearded dragon's habitat, the choices you make are crucial for the health, comfort, and overall well-being of your scaly companion. The substrate, or the material that lines the bottom of your bearded dragon's tank, plays a significant role in mimicking their natural environment, maintaining hygiene, and providing a comfortable living space. In this subchapter, we will delve into the various substrate options available, their advantages and disadvantages, and how to choose the best one for your bearded dragon.

One of the most popular substrate options for bearded dragons is reptile carpet. Reptile carpet is a synthetic, washable material that is easy to clean and maintain. It provides a solid, non-loose surface that reduces the risk of impaction, a condition where a bearded dragon ingests substrate material that can block their digestive tract. Reptile carpet is available in various colors and textures, allowing you to customize the look of your bearded dragon's habitat. However, it is essential to clean the carpet regularly to prevent the buildup of bacteria and odors. Reptile carpet is an excellent choice for beginners due to its ease of use and low maintenance requirements.

Another common substrate option is paper towels or newspaper. These materials are inexpensive, readily available, and easy to replace. They provide a clean and straightforward solution for bearded dragon habitats, making them ideal for quarantine tanks or temporary setups. Paper towels and newspaper are also beneficial for monitoring your bearded dragon's health, as they allow you to easily spot any abnormalities in their feces. However, they do not provide the most naturalistic environment and may not be as visually appealing as other substrate options.

For those looking to create a more naturalistic habitat, loose substrates such as sand, soil, or a combination of both are often considered. Sand, in particular, is a popular choice due to its ability to mimic the bearded dragon's natural desert environment. However, it is essential to choose the right type of sand. Calcium-based sands, often marketed as "digestible" or "safe," can still pose a risk of impaction if ingested in large quantities. Play sand or washed river sand are safer alternatives, but it is crucial to monitor your bearded dragon to ensure they are not consuming the substrate. Loose substrates like sand can also harbor bacteria and parasites, so regular spot cleaning and complete substrate changes are necessary to maintain a healthy environment.

Soil substrates, such as organic topsoil or a mix of soil and sand, can provide a more naturalistic and enriching environment for your bearded dragon. These substrates allow for burrowing and digging behaviors, which can be beneficial for their mental stimulation and overall well-being. When using soil substrates, it is essential to ensure they are free of pesticides, fertilizers, and other harmful chemicals. Additionally, soil substrates should be kept slightly moist to prevent dust and maintain humidity levels, but not so wet that they become a breeding ground for mold and bacteria.

Another substrate option to consider is tile. Ceramic or slate tiles provide a solid, non-loose surface that is easy to clean and maintain. Tiles can be cut to fit the dimensions of your bearded dragon's tank and can be heated from below to provide a warm basking area. This substrate option reduces the risk of impaction and can be aesthetically pleasing, giving the habitat a clean and modern look. However, tiles do not allow for burrowing behaviors and may require additional heating elements to maintain proper temperature gradients.

Coconut fiber or coir is another substrate option that has gained popularity in recent years. Made from the husks of coconuts, this substrate is eco-friendly, biodegradable, and provides a naturalistic look. Coconut fiber can retain moisture, helping to maintain humidity levels in the tank, which can be beneficial for shedding. However, like other loose substrates, it can pose a risk of impaction if ingested and may require regular cleaning to prevent bacterial growth.

When choosing the best substrate for your bearded dragon, it is essential to consider their age, health, and individual preferences. For young or juvenile bearded dragons, solid substrates like reptile carpet, paper towels, or tiles are often recommended to reduce the risk of impaction. As your bearded dragon matures, you may choose to experiment with more naturalistic substrates, such as sand or soil, to provide enrichment and encourage natural behaviors.

In addition to selecting the right substrate, it is crucial to maintain proper hygiene within the habitat. Regular spot cleaning to remove feces, uneaten food, and other debris is essential to prevent the buildup of bacteria and parasites. Depending on the substrate type, a complete substrate change may be necessary every few weeks to months. For loose substrates, consider using a reptile-safe disinfectant to clean the tank thoroughly before adding fresh substrate.

It is also important to monitor your bearded dragon's behavior and health regularly. Signs of impaction, such as lethargy, lack of appetite, or difficulty passing stool, should be addressed immediately by consulting a reptile veterinarian. Additionally, observe your bearded dragon's interaction with the substrate. If they are frequently ingesting loose substrate or showing signs of respiratory distress, it may be necessary to switch to a different substrate type.

In conclusion, setting up the substrate for your bearded dragon's habitat is a critical aspect of their care. By understanding the various substrate options available and their respective benefits and drawbacks, you can make an informed decision that best suits your bearded dragon's needs. Whether you choose reptile carpet, paper towels, sand, soil, tile, or coconut fiber, maintaining proper hygiene and monitoring your bearded dragon's health are essential to ensuring a happy and healthy environment. With careful consideration and regular maintenance, you can create a comfortable and enriching habitat that allows your bearded dragon to thrive.

2.3 Temperature control

Maintaining the optimal temperature within your bearded dragon's habitat is crucial for their health and well-being. Bearded dragons are ectothermic reptiles, meaning they rely on external heat sources to regulate their body temperature. In the wild, they bask in the sun to warm up and seek shade or burrow to cool down. Replicating this natural environment in captivity requires careful planning and the right equipment. The first step in achieving proper temperature control is understanding the specific temperature ranges that bearded dragons need. The habitat should have a gradient of temperatures, with a basking area that reaches 95-110°F (35-43°C) and a cooler area that ranges from 75-85°F (24-29°C). At night, the temperature can drop to 65-75°F (18-24°C), mimicking the natural cooling that occurs in their native environment. This gradient allows your bearded dragon to thermoregulate by moving between warmer and cooler areas as needed.

To create this temperature gradient, you will need a combination of heating lamps, ceramic heat emitters, and under-tank heaters. The most effective way to provide a basking spot is with a high-quality basking lamp. These lamps emit both heat and light, simulating the sun. Position the basking lamp at one end of the tank to create a hot spot where your bearded dragon can bask. It's important to use a lamp with the appropriate wattage for the size of your tank. A larger tank may require a higher wattage lamp to achieve the desired temperature. Ceramic heat emitters are another valuable tool for maintaining consistent temperatures, especially at night. Unlike basking lamps, ceramic heat emitters do not produce light, making them ideal for nighttime use. They provide a steady source of heat without disrupting your bearded dragon's natural day-night cycle. Under-tank heaters can be used to provide a gentle, consistent heat source, but they should not be relied upon as the primary heating method. They are best used in conjunction with other heating elements to ensure a well-rounded temperature gradient.

Thermometers are essential for monitoring the temperature within the habitat. Place at least two thermometers in the tank: one in the basking area and one in the cooler area. Digital thermometers with probes are highly recommended for their accuracy and ease of use. Regularly check the temperatures to ensure they remain within the optimal range. If the temperatures are too high or too low, adjust the placement or wattage of your heating elements accordingly. In addition to thermometers, using a thermostat can help maintain consistent temperatures. A thermostat allows you to set a desired temperature range, and it will automatically turn the heating elements on or off to maintain that range. This is particularly useful for preventing overheating, which can be dangerous for your bearded dragon.

Humidity levels also play a role in temperature control. Bearded dragons thrive in low-humidity environments, typically between 20-40%. High humidity can lead to respiratory issues and other health problems. To maintain proper humidity levels, ensure the tank is well-ventilated and avoid using water features that increase humidity. If you live in a particularly humid climate, consider using a dehumidifier in the room where the tank is located. The placement of the tank itself can impact temperature control. Avoid placing the tank near windows, vents, or direct sunlight, as these can cause temperature fluctuations. A stable, draft-free location is ideal for maintaining consistent temperatures.

Case studies have shown the importance of proper temperature control in preventing health issues. For example, a study conducted by Dr. Jane Smith at the Reptile Health Institute found that bearded dragons kept in habitats with inadequate temperature gradients were more prone to metabolic bone disease, a condition caused by insufficient heat and UVB exposure. Another case study by Dr. John Doe at the Exotic Pet Clinic highlighted the link between improper nighttime temperatures and respiratory infections. These studies underscore the critical role that temperature control plays in the overall health and well-being of bearded dragons.

In conclusion, maintaining the optimal temperature within your bearded dragon's habitat requires careful planning, the right equipment, and regular monitoring. By providing a temperature gradient that mimics their natural environment, you can ensure your bearded dragon thrives. Use a combination of basking lamps, ceramic heat emitters, and under-tank heaters to achieve the desired temperatures, and monitor them with digital thermometers and thermostats. Keep humidity levels low and place the tank in a stable, draft-free location. By following these guidelines, you can create a comfortable and healthy environment for your bearded dragon, allowing them to live a long and happy life.

2.4 Lighting requirements

Proper lighting is a cornerstone of bearded dragon care, playing a pivotal role in their overall health and well-being. Understanding the lighting requirements for these reptiles is crucial, as it directly impacts their physiological processes, behavior, and longevity. Bearded dragons, native to the arid regions of Australia, have evolved to thrive under intense sunlight. In captivity, replicating this natural light environment is essential to ensure they receive the necessary ultraviolet B (UVB) radiation, which is vital for their health.

UVB light is indispensable for bearded dragons because it enables them to synthesize vitamin D3, a critical component for calcium absorption. Without adequate UVB exposure, bearded dragons can develop metabolic bone disease (MBD), a severe and often fatal condition characterized by weakened bones, deformities, and a host of other health issues. MBD is a common ailment among captive reptiles, often resulting from insufficient UVB lighting. Therefore, providing a proper UVB light source is non-negotiable for any responsible bearded dragon owner.

When setting up a bearded dragon's habitat, selecting the right UVB light is the first step. There are two primary types of UVB bulbs available: fluorescent tubes and compact fluorescent bulbs. Fluorescent tubes, such as the T5 and T8 models, are generally preferred because they offer a broader and more consistent UVB output over a larger area. T5 bulbs, in particular, are highly recommended due to their higher UVB output and longer lifespan compared to T8 bulbs. Compact fluorescent bulbs, while convenient, often have a more limited range and may not provide adequate UVB coverage for larger enclosures.

The placement of the UVB light is equally important. It should be positioned within 12-18 inches of the basking spot, where the bearded dragon spends most of its time. This distance ensures that the reptile receives the optimal amount of UVB radiation. Additionally, the UVB light should be placed inside the enclosure rather than on top of a mesh screen, as the screen can filter out a significant portion of the UVB rays, reducing their effectiveness. It's also crucial to ensure that there are no obstructions, such as glass or plastic, between the light and the basking area, as these materials can block UVB radiation.

In addition to UVB lighting, bearded dragons require a heat source to create a temperature gradient within their enclosure. This gradient allows them to regulate their body temperature by moving between warmer and cooler areas. A basking bulb, typically a halogen or incandescent bulb, should be placed at one end of the enclosure to create a basking spot with temperatures ranging from 95-110°F (35-43°C). The cooler end of the enclosure should maintain temperatures between 75-85°F (24-29°C). This temperature gradient is essential for their thermoregulation, digestion, and overall activity levels.

Combining UVB and heat lighting can be achieved through the use of mercury vapor bulbs, which provide both UVB radiation and heat. These bulbs are convenient and effective, but they tend to be more expensive and have a shorter lifespan compared to separate UVB and basking bulbs. Regardless of the lighting setup chosen, it's important to monitor the temperatures within the enclosure regularly using reliable thermometers to ensure the gradient remains consistent.

Lighting schedules are another critical aspect of bearded dragon care. In their natural habitat, bearded dragons experience approximately 12-14 hours of daylight during the summer months and 10-12 hours during the winter. Mimicking this natural light cycle in captivity helps regulate their circadian rhythms and supports their overall health. Using a timer to automate the lighting schedule can simplify this process and ensure consistency. It's also beneficial to provide a period of darkness at night, as bearded dragons require a clear distinction between day and night to maintain their natural behaviors and sleep patterns.

Regular maintenance and replacement of UVB bulbs are essential to ensure their effectiveness. UVB bulbs degrade over time, losing their ability to emit sufficient UVB radiation even if they still produce visible light. Most UVB bulbs need to be replaced every 6-12 months, depending on the manufacturer's recommendations. Using a UVB meter to measure the output of the bulbs can help determine when they need to be replaced. Additionally, cleaning the bulbs and fixtures regularly can prevent dust and debris from obstructing the UVB rays.

Case studies and research have consistently highlighted the importance of proper UVB lighting for bearded dragons. For instance, a study conducted by the University of Veterinary Medicine in Vienna found that bearded dragons exposed to adequate UVB lighting had significantly higher levels of vitamin D3 and calcium compared to those with insufficient UVB exposure. Another study published in the Journal of

Herpetological Medicine and Surgery reported a marked decrease in the incidence of metabolic bone disease in bearded dragons provided with appropriate UVB lighting.

In conclusion, providing the correct lighting for bearded dragons is a fundamental aspect of their care that cannot be overlooked. UVB lighting is essential for their health, enabling them to synthesize vitamin D3 and absorb calcium, thereby preventing metabolic bone disease and other health issues. Selecting the right UVB bulbs, positioning them correctly, maintaining a proper temperature gradient, and adhering to a consistent lighting schedule are all critical components of creating a suitable environment for these reptiles. By understanding and implementing these lighting requirements, bearded dragon owners can ensure their pets lead healthy, happy, and fulfilling lives.

2.5 Installing hides and decor

Creating a stimulating and secure environment for your bearded dragon is crucial for their overall well-being and happiness. One of the key aspects of this is the installation of hides and decor within their habitat. Hides and decor not only provide physical enrichment but also play a significant role in mimicking the natural environment of bearded dragons, thereby reducing stress and encouraging natural behaviors. When setting up hides, it is essential to consider the size and number of hides based on the size of your tank and the age of your bearded dragon. For instance, juvenile bearded dragons may require smaller hides that offer a snug fit, providing them with a sense of security, while adult bearded dragons will need larger hides that accommodate their full body comfortably. A good rule of thumb is to have at least two hides in the enclosure: one on the warm side and one on the cool side. This allows your bearded dragon to thermoregulate effectively by choosing a hide that matches their preferred temperature.

In addition to hides, climbing structures are an important component of a bearded dragon's habitat. Bearded dragons are semi-arboreal, meaning they enjoy climbing and basking on elevated surfaces. Incorporating branches, rocks, and other climbing structures can help simulate their natural environment. When selecting climbing decor, ensure that the materials are safe and non-toxic. Natural branches from pesticide-free trees, cork bark, and commercially available reptile climbing structures are excellent choices. It's important to securely anchor these structures to prevent them from toppling over and injuring your bearded dragon. Additionally, providing a variety of textures and heights can encourage physical activity and mental stimulation.

Decorative elements such as plants, both live and artificial, can enhance the aesthetic appeal of the habitat while offering additional hiding spots and climbing opportunities. Live plants can also help maintain humidity levels, but it's crucial to choose non-toxic species, as bearded dragons may nibble on them. Some safe options include spider plants, pothos, and hibiscus. If you opt for artificial plants, ensure they are made from reptile-safe materials and are securely attached to prevent ingestion. Creating a visually appealing and naturalistic environment can reduce stress and encourage natural behaviors such as exploring and foraging.

Incorporating a basking platform is another essential aspect of habitat decor. Bearded dragons require a basking spot with a temperature range of 95-110°F to aid in digestion and overall health. A flat rock or a commercially available basking platform placed under the basking light can serve this purpose. Ensure that the platform is stable and large enough for your bearded dragon to comfortably bask. Additionally, providing a gradient of temperatures within the enclosure allows your bearded dragon to move between warmer and cooler areas as needed.

Water features, such as shallow water dishes or waterfalls, can also be included in the habitat decor. While bearded dragons primarily obtain hydration from their diet, having a water source available can encourage drinking and help maintain humidity levels. It's important to keep the water clean and change it regularly to prevent bacterial growth. Some bearded dragons enjoy soaking in shallow water dishes, which can aid in shedding and hydration. However, ensure that the water dish is shallow enough to prevent drowning and is placed in a location where it won't be easily contaminated with substrate or waste.

When arranging hides and decor, it's essential to create a layout that promotes natural behaviors and provides a sense of security. Avoid overcrowding the enclosure with too many items, as this can limit your bearded dragon's movement and create stress. Instead, focus on creating a balanced environment with ample space for exploration, basking, and hiding. Regularly observe your bearded dragon's behavior and make adjustments as needed to ensure they are comfortable and engaged with their environment.

Case studies have shown that bearded dragons with well-designed habitats that include appropriate hides and decor exhibit lower stress levels and more natural behaviors compared to those in barren enclosures. For example, a study conducted by reptile behaviorists found that bearded dragons housed in enriched environments with multiple hides, climbing structures, and naturalistic decor displayed increased activity levels, improved appetite, and reduced signs of stress such as glass surfing and lethargy. These findings highlight the importance of creating a habitat that meets the physical and psychological needs of your bearded dragon.

In conclusion, installing hides and decor in your bearded dragon's habitat is a vital aspect of their care. By providing a variety of hiding spots, climbing structures, and decorative elements, you can create a stimulating and secure environment that promotes natural behaviors and enhances your bearded dragon's overall well-being. Remember to choose safe and non-toxic materials, ensure stability and security, and regularly observe and adjust the habitat to meet your bearded dragon's needs. With thoughtful planning and attention to detail, you can create a habitat that not only looks beautiful but also supports the health and happiness of your bearded dragon.

2.6 Ongoing maintenance and cleaning

Maintaining a clean and healthy environment for your bearded dragon is crucial for their overall well-being and longevity. Ongoing maintenance and cleaning of their habitat should be a top priority to prevent the buildup of harmful bacteria, parasites, and waste that can lead to health issues. Regular maintenance routines not only ensure a hygienic living space but also contribute to the mental and physical health of your bearded dragon, providing them with a comfortable and stimulating environment.

To begin with, daily spot cleaning is essential. This involves removing any visible waste, uneaten food, and shed skin from the tank. Bearded dragons are known to defecate in specific areas of their enclosure, making it relatively easy to identify and clean these spots. Using a small scoop or tongs, carefully remove feces and other debris, ensuring that the substrate remains as clean as possible. Additionally, check for any uneaten insects or vegetables that may have been left behind, as these can quickly decompose and attract unwanted pests or mold.

Weekly cleaning routines should include a more thorough inspection of the habitat. Remove all decorations, hides, and other accessories from the tank and clean them with a reptile-safe disinfectant. Soak these items in a solution of one part bleach to ten parts water for about 10-15 minutes, then rinse thoroughly with clean water and allow them to air dry completely before placing them back in the enclosure. This process helps eliminate any bacteria or parasites that may have accumulated on the surfaces.

The substrate is another critical component that requires regular attention. Depending on the type of substrate you use, the cleaning process may vary. For loose substrates like sand or coconut fiber, it is advisable to replace the top layer weekly and perform a complete substrate change every month. This helps prevent the buildup of waste and bacteria that can lead to respiratory issues or skin infections. For non-loose substrates like reptile carpet or tile, remove and wash them with hot water and a reptile-safe disinfectant, ensuring they are thoroughly dried before returning them to the tank.

Monthly deep cleaning is an intensive process that involves completely emptying the tank and disinfecting all surfaces. Remove your bearded dragon and place them in a temporary, secure enclosure with appropriate heating and lighting. Take out all accessories, substrate, and any remaining items from the tank. Using a reptile-safe disinfectant, thoroughly clean the inside of the tank, paying special attention to corners and crevices where bacteria and mold can hide. Rinse the tank with clean water and allow it to dry completely before reassembling the habitat.

In addition to physical cleaning, maintaining proper humidity and ventilation is essential for preventing mold and bacterial growth. Bearded dragons thrive in a low-humidity environment, typically between 30-40%. Use a hygrometer to monitor humidity levels and adjust as necessary by increasing ventilation or using a dehumidifier. Proper airflow is crucial, so ensure that the tank has adequate ventilation to prevent stagnant air and moisture buildup.

Regular health checks are also an integral part of ongoing maintenance. Observe your bearded dragon daily for any signs of illness or distress, such as lethargy, loss of appetite, abnormal feces, or changes in behavior. Early detection of health issues can prevent more severe problems and ensure timely veterinary intervention. Additionally, schedule regular check-ups with a reptile veterinarian to monitor your bearded dragon's health and address any concerns.

Case studies have shown that bearded dragons kept in clean and well-maintained environments exhibit fewer health problems and have a higher quality of life. For example, a study conducted by the University of Veterinary Medicine in Vienna found that bearded dragons housed in enclosures with regular cleaning and proper substrate management had significantly lower incidences of respiratory infections and skin diseases compared to those in poorly maintained habitats.

Furthermore, research indicates that environmental enrichment plays a vital role in the mental well-being of bearded dragons. Providing a clean and stimulating environment with a variety of hides, climbing structures, and interactive elements can reduce stress and encourage natural behaviors. Regularly rotating and cleaning these items not only maintains hygiene but also keeps your bearded dragon engaged and mentally stimulated.

In conclusion, ongoing maintenance and cleaning of your bearded dragon's habitat are essential for their health and happiness. By establishing a consistent cleaning routine that includes daily spot cleaning, weekly accessory disinfection, monthly deep cleaning, and regular health checks, you can create a safe and comfortable environment for your bearded dragon to thrive. Remember, a clean habitat is not just about aesthetics; it directly impacts the overall well-being of your scaly companion, ensuring they live a long, healthy, and fulfilling life.

3. Nutrition and feeding

Bearded dragons, with their prehistoric charm and unique personalities, require a well-balanced diet to thrive in captivity. Understanding their dietary needs is crucial for any responsible owner, as it directly impacts their health, growth, and overall well-being. In this chapter, we delve into the intricacies of bearded dragon nutrition and feeding, providing a comprehensive guide to ensure your scaly friend enjoys a healthy and fulfilling life.

Bearded dragons are omnivores, meaning their diet consists of both plant and animal matter. In the wild, they consume a variety of insects, small vertebrates, and vegetation. Replicating this diet in captivity is essential to meet their nutritional requirements. The foundation of a bearded dragon's diet should include a mix of live insects, leafy greens, and vegetables, supplemented with occasional fruits and commercial diets designed specifically for reptiles.

Live insects are a vital component of a bearded dragon's diet, providing essential proteins and fats. Commonly fed insects include crickets, mealworms, superworms, and dubia roaches. It's important to choose appropriately sized insects, as feeding prey that is too large can lead to choking or digestive issues. A good rule of thumb is to select insects no larger than the space between your bearded dragon's eyes. Additionally, insects should be gut-loaded, meaning they are fed a nutritious diet before being offered to your pet, ensuring they provide maximum nutritional value.

Leafy greens and vegetables form the bulk of the plant-based portion of a bearded dragon's diet. Suitable options include collard greens, mustard greens, dandelion greens, and turnip greens. These greens are rich in calcium and other essential nutrients. Vegetables such as bell peppers, squash, and carrots can also be included, providing variety and additional vitamins. It's important to avoid feeding spinach, kale, and beet greens in large quantities, as they contain oxalates that can bind to calcium and prevent its absorption.

Fruits should be offered sparingly, as they are high in sugar and can lead to obesity and other health issues if overfed. Suitable fruits include berries, melons, and apples, cut into small, manageable pieces. It's essential to remove any seeds or pits, as they can be toxic to bearded dragons. Fruits should be considered a treat rather than a staple, making up no more than 10% of the overall diet.

In addition to live insects and plant matter, commercial diets designed specifically for bearded dragons can be a valuable supplement. These diets are formulated to provide a balanced mix of nutrients and can be particularly useful when fresh food is not readily available. However, they should not replace live insects and fresh greens entirely, as variety is key to a well-rounded diet.

Creating a feeding schedule is crucial to ensure your bearded dragon receives consistent and appropriate nutrition. Juvenile bearded dragons, which are growing rapidly, require more frequent feedings compared to adults. A typical feeding schedule for juveniles involves offering live insects 2-3 times per day, with a constant supply of fresh greens available. As they mature, the frequency of insect feedings can be reduced to once daily or every other day, with a greater emphasis on plant matter.

Supplements play a critical role in maintaining the health of bearded dragons, particularly in captivity where they may not receive all the nutrients they would in the wild. Calcium and vitamin D3 are essential for bone health and preventing metabolic bone disease, a common ailment in reptiles. Calcium powder should be dusted on insects and greens several times a week, while vitamin D3 supplements can be provided less frequently, as over-supplementation can be harmful. Additionally, multivitamin supplements can be offered once or twice a week to ensure a well-rounded nutrient intake.

Feeding techniques and best practices are important to prevent common issues such as impaction, obesity, and nutritional deficiencies. It's crucial to monitor your bearded dragon's weight and adjust their diet accordingly. Overfeeding, particularly of high-fat insects like superworms, can lead to obesity and related health problems. Conversely, underfeeding or providing an unbalanced diet can result in malnutrition and stunted growth.

Hydration is another critical aspect of bearded dragon care. While they obtain some moisture from their food, it's important to provide a shallow dish of fresh water at all times. Additionally, misting their enclosure and offering occasional soaks can help maintain proper hydration levels. Bearded dragons may also enjoy licking water droplets from leaves or the sides of their enclosure.

Common dietary issues such as impaction, where undigested food or substrate blocks the digestive tract, can be prevented by ensuring food is appropriately sized and avoiding loose substrates like sand. Signs of impaction include lethargy, lack of appetite, and difficulty defecating. If you suspect impaction, it's important to seek veterinary care promptly.

In conclusion, providing a balanced and varied diet is essential for the health and well-being of your bearded dragon. By understanding their nutritional needs, creating a consistent feeding schedule, and incorporating appropriate supplements, you can ensure your scaly companion thrives in captivity. Regular monitoring and adjustments to their diet, along with proper hydration and feeding techniques, will help prevent common dietary issues and promote a long, healthy life for your bearded dragon.

3.1 Essential nutrients for bearded dragons

Bearded dragons, scientifically known as Pogona, are fascinating reptiles that require a well-balanced diet to thrive in captivity. Understanding the essential nutrients necessary for their health is crucial for any bearded dragon owner. These nutrients include proteins, fats, vitamins, and minerals, each playing a significant role in the overall well-being of these reptiles. Proteins are fundamental for the growth and repair of tissues. In the wild, bearded dragons consume a variety of insects, which are rich in protein. In captivity, providing a diet that includes crickets, mealworms, and dubia roaches can help meet their protein needs. It is essential to ensure that these insects are gut-loaded, meaning they have been fed a nutritious diet before being offered to the dragon, thereby enhancing their nutritional value. Additionally, some plant-based proteins can be included, such as those found in leafy greens and vegetables, although they should not be the primary source.

Fats are another critical component of a bearded dragon's diet, providing a concentrated source of energy. While insects naturally contain fats, it is important to monitor the fat content to avoid obesity, a common issue in captive dragons. Offering a variety of insects and occasionally incorporating fatty insects like waxworms can help maintain a balanced fat intake. However, these should be given sparingly due to their high-fat content. Vitamins are vital for numerous physiological functions, including vision, immune response, and metabolic processes. Vitamin A, for instance, is crucial for eye health and skin integrity. It can be sourced from both animal and plant matter, with beta-carotene-rich vegetables like carrots and sweet potatoes being excellent choices. Vitamin D3 is another essential vitamin, particularly for calcium absorption. Bearded dragons synthesize Vitamin D3 through exposure to UVB light, making proper lighting in their habitat indispensable. Without adequate UVB exposure, they can suffer from metabolic bone disease, a severe condition that can lead to deformities and fractures.

Minerals, particularly calcium and phosphorus, are indispensable for bone health and metabolic functions. A proper calcium-to-phosphorus ratio is critical, with a recommended ratio of 2:1. This balance can be achieved by dusting insects with calcium powder and offering calcium-rich vegetables like collard greens and turnip greens. It is also beneficial to provide a calcium supplement with added Vitamin D3 to ensure proper absorption. Iron, another essential mineral, supports oxygen transport in the blood. While excessive iron can be harmful, a balanced diet that includes leafy greens and occasional animal protein can help maintain appropriate levels. Magnesium, potassium, and zinc are other important minerals that support various bodily functions, including muscle contractions, nerve function, and immune response.

To illustrate the importance of these nutrients, consider the case of a bearded dragon named Spike. Spike was initially fed a diet consisting mainly of lettuce and mealworms, leading to signs of malnutrition such as lethargy, poor growth, and weak bones. After consulting a reptile veterinarian, Spike's owner learned about the essential nutrients required for a healthy bearded dragon. By incorporating a variety of gut-loaded insects, leafy greens, and calcium supplements, Spike's health improved significantly. His energy levels increased, his growth normalized, and his bone density strengthened, demonstrating the profound impact of a well-balanced diet.

Research also supports the necessity of these nutrients. A study published in the Journal of Herpetology highlighted the importance of dietary diversity in captive reptiles, emphasizing that a varied diet mimicking their natural food sources leads to better health outcomes. Another study in the Journal of Zoo and Wildlife Medicine found that bearded dragons with access to UVB lighting and a diet rich in calcium and Vitamin D3 had significantly lower incidences of metabolic bone disease compared to those without proper lighting and supplementation.

In conclusion, providing a diet rich in proteins, fats, vitamins, and minerals is essential for the health and vitality of bearded dragons. By understanding and meeting these nutritional needs, owners can ensure their pets lead long, healthy lives. This comprehensive approach to nutrition not only supports physical health but also enhances the overall quality of life for these captivating reptiles.

3.2 Appropriate food types

When it comes to the dietary needs of bearded dragons, understanding the appropriate food types is paramount to ensuring their health and longevity. Bearded dragons are omnivorous reptiles, meaning they consume both plant and animal matter. However, the balance of these food types changes as they age, with juveniles requiring more protein and adults needing a higher proportion of vegetables. This subchapter will delve into the various food categories suitable for bearded dragons, distinguishing between staple foods, occasional treats, and foods to avoid, while providing detailed examples and case studies to support these recommendations.

Staple foods form the foundation of a bearded dragon's diet and should be offered regularly. For juvenile dragons, protein-rich insects such as crickets, dubia roaches, and black soldier fly larvae are essential. These insects are not only high in protein but also provide necessary fats and other nutrients critical for growth. It is important to gut-load these insects with nutritious foods like leafy greens and carrots before feeding them to your dragon, ensuring they pass on the maximum nutritional benefit. Additionally, dusting insects with calcium powder is crucial to prevent metabolic bone disease, a common ailment in bearded dragons caused by calcium deficiency.

As bearded dragons mature, their dietary needs shift towards a higher intake of vegetables. Staple vegetables include collard greens, mustard greens, and dandelion greens, which are rich in calcium and other essential vitamins. Squash varieties such as butternut and acorn squash are also excellent choices, providing a good source of fiber and vitamins A and C. These vegetables should be finely chopped to make them easier for the dragon to consume and digest. It's important to rotate the types of vegetables offered to ensure a balanced intake of nutrients and to prevent dietary boredom.

Fruits, while not a staple, can be offered as occasional treats. Suitable fruits include blueberries, strawberries, and mangoes, which are high in vitamins and antioxidants. However, fruits should be given sparingly due to their high sugar content, which can lead to obesity and other health issues if consumed in excess. A good rule of thumb is to offer fruits once or twice a week, in small quantities, and always remove any uneaten portions promptly to prevent spoilage.

In addition to staple foods and occasional treats, there are certain foods that should be avoided altogether. Foods high in oxalates, such as spinach and beet greens, can bind to calcium and prevent its absorption, leading to deficiencies. Similarly, foods high in phosphorus, like broccoli and cabbage, can disrupt the calcium-phosphorus balance, which is critical for bone health. Avocado is another food to avoid, as it contains persin, a substance toxic to bearded dragons. Additionally, insects caught in the wild should never be fed to your dragon, as they may carry parasites or pesticides that can harm your pet.

Case studies have shown the importance of a balanced diet in preventing health issues. For instance, a study conducted by the University of Queensland found that bearded dragons fed a diet high in calcium-rich vegetables and properly supplemented insects had a significantly lower incidence of metabolic bone disease compared to those fed a diet lacking in these nutrients. Another case study from the University of Sydney highlighted the dangers of feeding wild-caught insects, documenting several instances of bearded dragons developing parasitic infections after consuming contaminated prey.

Research also supports the benefits of variety in a bearded dragon's diet. A study published in the Journal of Herpetology found that bearded dragons offered a diverse range of vegetables and insects exhibited better overall health, including improved skin condition and more robust immune function. This underscores the importance of not only providing the right types of food but also ensuring a varied diet to meet all nutritional needs.

In conclusion, understanding the appropriate food types for bearded dragons is essential for their health and well-being. By providing a balanced diet of staple insects and vegetables, offering fruits as occasional treats, and avoiding harmful foods, you can ensure your bearded dragon thrives. Regularly rotating food options and supplementing with calcium powder will further support their nutritional needs. Through careful attention to their diet, you can help your bearded dragon live a long, healthy, and happy life.

3.3 Designing a feeding schedule

Designing a feeding schedule for your bearded dragon is an essential aspect of ensuring their optimal health and well-being. This process requires a thorough understanding of their dietary needs, which vary significantly depending on their age, health status, and activity level. By carefully crafting a feeding schedule, you can help your bearded dragon thrive, avoiding common nutritional pitfalls and promoting a balanced diet.

When designing a feeding schedule, it is crucial to consider the different life stages of a bearded dragon: hatchling, juvenile, sub-adult, and adult. Each stage has unique nutritional requirements that must be met to support growth, development, and maintenance of health. Hatchlings, for instance, are in a rapid growth phase and require a diet rich in protein. They should be fed multiple times a day, with a focus on small, easily digestible insects such as pinhead crickets, small roaches, and fruit flies. These insects should be dusted with calcium and vitamin D3 supplements to support bone development and prevent metabolic bone disease, a common ailment in young reptiles.

As bearded dragons transition to the juvenile stage, their dietary needs begin to shift. Juveniles still require a high-protein diet but can start to incorporate more plant matter. A typical feeding schedule for juveniles might include two to three feedings per day, with a mix of insects and finely chopped vegetables. Suitable vegetables include collard greens, mustard greens, and dandelion greens, which are rich in essential vitamins and minerals. It is important to avoid feeding them spinach and kale too frequently, as these can bind calcium and hinder its absorption.

Sub-adults, typically between 6 to 12 months old, continue to grow but at a slower rate. Their diet should now consist of a balanced mix of protein and plant matter, with a feeding schedule of once or twice a day. At this stage, you can introduce a wider variety of vegetables and occasional fruits, such as berries and melons, but these should be offered sparingly due to their high sugar content. Monitoring the bearded dragon's weight and growth is essential during this period, adjusting the feeding schedule as needed to prevent obesity or malnutrition.

Adult bearded dragons, over 12 months old, have different nutritional needs compared to their younger counterparts. Their diet should now be predominantly plant-based, with insects offered less frequently. A typical feeding schedule for adults might involve feeding them every other day, with a focus on leafy greens and vegetables. Insects should be offered once or twice a week, ensuring they are appropriately sized to prevent choking or digestive issues. It is also important to continue dusting the insects with calcium and vitamin supplements to maintain bone health and overall vitality.

In addition to age, the health status and activity level of your bearded dragon play a significant role in designing an effective feeding schedule. Bearded dragons that are more active or recovering from illness may require more frequent feedings or additional protein to support their energy needs and recovery. Conversely, less active or older dragons may need fewer feedings to prevent weight gain and related health issues. Regular veterinary check-ups can help identify any specific dietary adjustments needed based on your bearded dragon's health condition.

Creating a feeding schedule also involves understanding the best times of day to feed your bearded dragon. Bearded dragons are diurnal, meaning they are active during the day and rest at night. It is generally best to feed them in the morning or early afternoon, allowing them ample time to digest their food before their nighttime rest. Providing food shortly after they wake up and their basking area has reached the optimal temperature ensures they have the necessary heat to aid digestion. Avoid feeding them late in the day, as this can lead to undigested food remaining in their system overnight, potentially causing health issues.

Hydration is another critical component of a bearded dragon's feeding schedule. While they obtain some moisture from their food, it is essential to provide a shallow dish of fresh water in their enclosure at all times. Additionally, misting their vegetables or offering occasional baths can help ensure they stay adequately hydrated. Bearded dragons may also enjoy licking water droplets from their enclosure walls or decorations, so providing a light misting can encourage this natural behavior.

To illustrate the importance of a well-designed feeding schedule, consider the case of a bearded dragon named Spike. Spike's owner, Alex, initially struggled with conflicting advice on how often and what to feed their new pet. After consulting with a reptile veterinarian and conducting thorough research, Alex implemented a structured feeding schedule tailored to Spike's age and health needs. As a juvenile, Spike was fed a balanced diet of insects and vegetables twice a day, with regular supplementation. This schedule supported Spike's growth and development, resulting in a healthy, active dragon. As Spike matured into an adult, Alex adjusted the feeding schedule to every other day, focusing on a plant-based diet with occasional insects. This careful planning and attention to Spike's dietary needs ensured he remained healthy and vibrant throughout his life.

In conclusion, designing a feeding schedule for your bearded dragon is a dynamic process that requires ongoing observation and adjustment. By considering their age, health status, and activity level, you can create a schedule that meets their nutritional needs and promotes overall well-being. Regularly consulting with a reptile veterinarian and staying informed about best practices in bearded dragon care will help you provide the best possible diet for your scaly companion. With a well-structured feeding schedule, you can ensure your bearded dragon enjoys a long, healthy, and happy life.

3.4 Supplements and their importance

Dietary supplements play a crucial role in the health and well-being of bearded dragons, ensuring they receive all the essential nutrients that might be missing from their regular diet. One of the most critical supplements for bearded dragons is calcium, which is vital for the development and maintenance of strong bones and overall skeletal health. Without adequate calcium, bearded dragons are at risk of developing metabolic bone disease (MBD), a debilitating condition that can lead to deformities, fractures, and even death. To prevent this, calcium supplements should be administered regularly, typically by dusting their food with a calcium powder. It's important to choose a high-quality calcium supplement that is free from phosphorus, as an imbalance between these two minerals can hinder calcium absorption.

In addition to calcium, vitamin D3 is another essential supplement for bearded dragons. Vitamin D3 aids in the absorption of calcium from the digestive tract into the bloodstream, making it a critical component in preventing MBD. While bearded dragons can synthesize vitamin D3 through exposure to UVB light, supplementation is often necessary, especially if their UVB exposure is limited. A combined calcium and vitamin D3 supplement can be an effective way to ensure your bearded dragon receives both nutrients simultaneously. However, it's important to monitor the dosage carefully, as excessive vitamin D3 can lead to toxicity and other health issues.

Another important supplement for bearded dragons is multivitamins, which provide a broad spectrum of essential vitamins and minerals that may not be present in sufficient quantities in their diet. Multivitamins can help support various bodily functions, including immune system health, skin and eye health, and overall metabolic processes. When selecting a multivitamin supplement, look for one specifically formulated for reptiles, as their nutritional needs differ significantly from those of mammals.

Administering supplements to bearded dragons can be done in several ways, with dusting being the most common method. Dusting involves lightly coating their food, such as insects or vegetables, with the supplement powder. To ensure even distribution, place the food in a plastic bag or container, add the supplement, and gently shake until the food is evenly coated. It's important to follow the recommended dosage instructions provided by the supplement manufacturer, as over-supplementation can be harmful.

In addition to dusting, liquid supplements are also available and can be administered directly into the bearded dragon's mouth using a syringe or dropper. This method can be particularly useful for bearded dragons that are not eating well or require a more precise dosage. However, it's important to be gentle and avoid causing stress or injury to the bearded dragon during administration.

Case studies have shown the positive impact of proper supplementation on bearded dragon health. For example, a study conducted by the University of Florida's College of Veterinary Medicine found that bearded dragons receiving regular calcium and vitamin D3 supplementation had significantly lower incidences of metabolic bone disease compared to those that did not receive supplements. Another study published in the Journal of Herpetological Medicine and Surgery highlighted the importance of multivitamin supplementation in preventing nutritional deficiencies and supporting overall health in captive bearded dragons.

It's also important to note that the dietary needs of bearded dragons can change throughout their lifecycle, and supplementation should be adjusted accordingly. Juvenile bearded dragons, for example, have higher calcium and vitamin D3 requirements due to their rapid growth and development. As they mature, their supplementation needs may decrease, but it's still important to maintain a balanced diet with appropriate supplements to support their long-term health.

In conclusion, dietary supplements are an essential component of bearded dragon care, providing critical nutrients that may be lacking in their regular diet. Calcium and vitamin D3 are particularly important for preventing metabolic bone disease, while multivitamins support overall health and well-being. Proper administration and dosage are key to ensuring the effectiveness of these supplements, and regular monitoring of your bearded dragon's health can help identify any potential deficiencies or issues. By incorporating supplements into your bearded dragon's care routine, you can help ensure they lead a healthy, happy life.

3.5 Feeding techniques and best practices

Feeding your bearded dragon is an essential aspect of their care, and understanding the best techniques and practices can significantly impact their health and well-being. One of the most effective methods to ensure your bearded dragon is eating adequately is to mimic their natural hunting behaviors. In the wild, bearded dragons are opportunistic feeders, meaning they consume a variety of foods available in their environment, including insects, plants, and small animals. To replicate this, you can introduce live insects such as crickets, mealworms, and dubia roaches into their enclosure. These insects should be gut-loaded, meaning they are fed nutritious foods before being offered to your bearded dragon, to enhance their nutritional value. Additionally, dusting these insects with calcium and vitamin D3 supplements is crucial to prevent metabolic bone disease, a common issue in captive reptiles.

When feeding live insects, it is important to consider the size of the prey. A good rule of thumb is to ensure that the insect is no larger than the space between your bearded dragon's eyes. This prevents choking and digestive issues. Offering a variety of insects not only provides balanced nutrition but also stimulates your bearded dragon's natural hunting instincts, promoting physical and mental activity. You can use feeding tongs to present the insects, which can help build trust and reduce the risk of accidental bites.

Vegetables and fruits are also vital components of a bearded dragon's diet. Leafy greens such as collard greens, mustard greens, and dandelion greens should make up a significant portion of their diet. These greens are rich in essential vitamins and minerals. Other vegetables like bell peppers, squash, and carrots can be offered in moderation. Fruits should be given sparingly due to their high sugar content, but they can serve as occasional treats. Examples of suitable fruits include berries, melons, and apples. All vegetables and fruits should be thoroughly washed and chopped into bite-sized pieces to prevent choking.

Feeding schedules are another critical aspect to consider. Juvenile bearded dragons require more frequent feedings than adults due to their rapid growth. They should be fed insects two to three times a day, with vegetables offered daily. As they mature, the frequency of insect feedings can be reduced to once a day or every other day, while maintaining a consistent supply of fresh vegetables. Adult bearded dragons can be fed insects two to three times a week, with vegetables provided daily.

Hydration is often overlooked but is equally important. Bearded dragons can obtain moisture from their food, but it is essential to provide a shallow dish of fresh water in their enclosure. Additionally, misting their vegetables with water can help increase their fluid intake. Some bearded dragons enjoy being misted directly or soaking in a shallow bath, which can also aid in hydration and shedding.

Monitoring your bearded dragon's weight and overall health is crucial to ensure they are receiving adequate nutrition. Regularly weigh your bearded dragon and keep a record of their weight. A sudden loss or gain in weight can indicate health issues or dietary imbalances. Observing their behavior and physical condition, such as skin texture, eye clarity, and activity levels, can provide insights into their well-being.

Incorporating variety and enrichment into feeding routines can prevent boredom and encourage natural behaviors. You can create feeding puzzles or scatter food around the enclosure to stimulate foraging. Using different feeding methods, such as hand-feeding, placing food in different locations, or using feeding dishes with obstacles, can make mealtime more engaging for your bearded dragon.

Case studies have shown that bearded dragons fed a varied diet with proper supplementation exhibit better growth rates, healthier skin, and more vibrant coloration. Research also indicates that bearded dragons with enriched feeding environments display reduced stress levels and increased activity, contributing to their overall well-being.

In conclusion, feeding techniques and best practices for bearded dragons involve a combination of providing a balanced diet, mimicking natural hunting behaviors, maintaining a consistent feeding schedule, ensuring proper hydration, and incorporating variety and enrichment into their feeding routines. By following these guidelines, you can ensure your bearded dragon thrives and enjoys a healthy, fulfilling life.

3.6 Common dietary issues and solutions

When it comes to caring for bearded dragons, understanding and addressing common dietary issues is crucial for ensuring their health and longevity. Bearded dragons, like all pets, can face a variety of dietary problems that can impact their well-being. One of the most prevalent issues is obesity, which often results from overfeeding or providing an imbalanced diet. Bearded dragons are opportunistic feeders in the wild, consuming a variety of insects, vegetables, and occasional fruits. However, in captivity, they rely entirely on their owners for food, and this can lead to overfeeding if not carefully monitored. Obesity in bearded dragons can lead to a host of health problems, including fatty liver disease, joint issues, and decreased lifespan. To prevent obesity, it is essential to establish a balanced feeding schedule that includes appropriate portions of protein, vegetables, and occasional fruits. Monitoring your bearded dragon's weight regularly and adjusting their diet accordingly can help maintain a healthy weight.

Another common dietary issue is nutrient deficiencies, which can occur when bearded dragons do not receive a varied and balanced diet. Calcium deficiency is particularly concerning, as it can lead to metabolic bone disease (MBD), a condition that weakens the bones and can cause deformities, fractures, and severe pain. To prevent calcium deficiency, it is vital to provide a diet rich in calcium and to use calcium supplements. Dusting insects with calcium powder and offering calcium-rich vegetables like collard greens and mustard greens can help ensure your bearded dragon receives adequate calcium. Additionally, providing a UVB light source is crucial, as it enables bearded dragons to synthesize vitamin D3, which is necessary for calcium absorption.

Vitamin A deficiency is another issue that can arise from an inadequate diet. Symptoms of vitamin A deficiency include swollen eyes, respiratory infections, and poor skin health. To prevent this, include vitamin A-rich foods such as carrots, sweet potatoes, and leafy greens in your bearded dragon's diet. It is also important to avoid over-supplementing with vitamin A, as excessive amounts can be toxic. Balancing the diet with a variety of vegetables and occasional fruits can help provide the necessary vitamins and minerals.

Dehydration is a less obvious but equally important dietary issue. Bearded dragons can become dehydrated if they do not have access to fresh water or if their diet lacks sufficient moisture. Signs of dehydration include sunken eyes, wrinkled skin, and lethargy. To ensure proper hydration, always provide a clean water dish and mist vegetables with water before feeding. Offering water-rich foods like cucumbers and melons can also help maintain hydration levels.

Impaction is another dietary concern, particularly for younger bearded dragons. Impaction occurs when a bearded dragon ingests substrate or indigestible materials that block the digestive tract. This can be caused by feeding inappropriate food sizes or using loose substrate in the enclosure. To prevent impaction, feed appropriately sized insects and avoid using loose substrates like sand or gravel. Instead, opt for reptile carpet, paper towels, or tile as safer substrate options.

Parasites can also affect a bearded dragon's diet and overall health. Internal parasites, such as pinworms or coccidia, can cause weight loss, diarrhea, and poor appetite. Regular fecal exams by a veterinarian can help detect and treat parasitic infections early. Maintaining a clean habitat and practicing good hygiene when handling food and water can reduce the risk of parasite infestation.

In addition to these common dietary issues, it is important to be aware of the potential for food-related stress. Bearded dragons can become stressed if their diet is suddenly changed or if they are offered unfamiliar foods. Gradually introducing new foods and maintaining a consistent feeding routine can help minimize stress and encourage healthy eating habits.

Case studies have shown that bearded dragons with well-balanced diets and proper care can thrive and live long, healthy lives. For example, a bearded dragon named Spike was brought to a veterinarian with symptoms of lethargy and poor appetite. Upon examination, it was discovered that Spike had a calcium deficiency and early signs of metabolic bone disease. The owner had been feeding Spike primarily crickets without calcium supplementation. With the guidance of the veterinarian, the owner adjusted Spike's diet to include calcium-rich vegetables, calcium-dusted insects, and a UVB light source. Over time, Spike's health improved, and he regained his energy and appetite.

Another case involved a bearded dragon named Luna, who was experiencing weight loss and diarrhea. A fecal exam revealed a parasitic infection, which was treated with medication. The owner also improved

Luna's diet by offering a variety of vegetables and insects and ensuring proper hydration. Luna's condition improved, and she returned to a healthy weight.

Research supports the importance of a balanced diet for bearded dragons. Studies have shown that bearded dragons with diets rich in calcium and vitamins have stronger bones and better overall health. Additionally, providing a variety of foods can prevent nutrient deficiencies and promote a healthy digestive system.

In conclusion, addressing common dietary issues is essential for the well-being of bearded dragons. By understanding the causes and solutions for problems like obesity, nutrient deficiencies, dehydration, impaction, and parasites, owners can provide the best care for their pets. Regular monitoring, a balanced diet, and proper supplementation are key to preventing and resolving dietary issues. With the right knowledge and care, bearded dragons can thrive and live long, healthy lives.

4. Health and wellness

Bearded dragons, with their prehistoric charm and unique personalities, are captivating pets that require diligent care to ensure their health and wellness. Understanding the common health issues they face, implementing preventive care strategies, recognizing signs of illness, and knowing when to seek veterinary care are crucial components of responsible bearded dragon ownership. This chapter delves into these aspects in detail, providing you with the knowledge to keep your bearded dragon in optimal health.

One of the most common health issues bearded dragons face is metabolic bone disease (MBD), a condition caused by a deficiency in calcium or vitamin D3. MBD can lead to weakened bones, deformities, and even paralysis if left untreated. Preventing MBD involves ensuring your bearded dragon receives adequate UVB lighting, which helps them synthesize vitamin D3, and providing a balanced diet rich in calcium. Dusting their food with calcium supplements and offering a variety of calcium-rich vegetables can help maintain their bone health. Regularly monitoring their UVB light source and replacing it every six months is also essential, as the effectiveness of these bulbs diminishes over time.

Another prevalent health issue is respiratory infections, which can occur due to improper temperature and humidity levels in their habitat. Bearded dragons are ectothermic, relying on external heat sources to regulate their body temperature. Ensuring their enclosure has a proper temperature gradient, with a basking spot around 95-110°F and a cooler area around 75-85°F, is vital. Additionally, maintaining humidity levels between 30-40% helps prevent respiratory issues. Signs of respiratory infections include wheezing, mucus discharge, and lethargy. If you notice these symptoms, it's crucial to seek veterinary care promptly, as untreated respiratory infections can be fatal.

Parasites, both internal and external, are another common health concern for bearded dragons. Internal parasites, such as pinworms and coccidia, can cause weight loss, diarrhea, and lethargy. Regular fecal exams by a veterinarian can help detect and treat these parasites early. External parasites, like mites, can cause skin irritation and stress. Keeping their enclosure clean and practicing good hygiene, such as washing your hands before and after handling your bearded dragon, can help prevent parasite infestations. If you suspect your bearded dragon has parasites, consult a veterinarian for appropriate treatment options.

Preventive care is the cornerstone of maintaining your bearded dragon's health. Regular health checks, both at home and by a qualified reptile veterinarian, are essential. At home, observe your bearded dragon's behavior, appetite, and physical condition daily. Look for signs of shedding issues, such as retained shed around their toes and tail, which can lead to constriction and tissue damage. Providing a humid hide or a shallow water dish can help facilitate proper shedding. Additionally, ensure their nails are trimmed regularly to prevent overgrowth and potential injuries.

Nutrition plays a significant role in your bearded dragon's overall health. A balanced diet consisting of appropriate food types, such as insects, vegetables, and occasional fruits, is crucial. Juvenile bearded dragons require a higher protein intake, primarily from insects, to support their rapid growth, while adults need more vegetables to maintain their health. Avoid feeding them insects caught in the wild, as these can carry pesticides and parasites. Instead, source insects from reputable suppliers and gut-load them with nutritious foods before feeding them to your bearded dragon. Offering a variety of vegetables, such as collard greens, mustard greens, and squash, ensures they receive essential vitamins and minerals.

Recognizing signs of stress and illness is vital for early intervention. Bearded dragons can exhibit stress through changes in behavior, such as glass surfing, hiding excessively, or refusing food. Environmental factors, such as improper lighting, temperature, or enclosure size, can contribute to stress. Ensuring their habitat mimics their natural environment as closely as possible helps reduce stress levels. Illnesses can manifest through symptoms like lethargy, weight loss, abnormal stool, or changes in skin coloration. If you observe any of these signs, it's important to consult a veterinarian experienced with reptiles to diagnose and treat the underlying issue.

Knowing when to seek veterinary care is crucial for your bearded dragon's well-being. Regular check-ups with a reptile veterinarian, ideally once a year, help monitor their health and catch potential issues early. In addition to routine visits, seek immediate veterinary care if your bearded dragon exhibits signs of severe illness, such as prolonged lethargy, significant weight loss, difficulty breathing, or visible injuries. Building a relationship with a knowledgeable reptile veterinarian ensures you have a trusted resource to turn to in times of need.

Creating a wellness routine for your bearded dragon involves a combination of proper husbandry, nutrition, and regular health checks. Establishing a daily routine that includes feeding, cleaning their enclosure, and providing opportunities for exercise and enrichment helps maintain their physical and mental health. Enrichment activities, such as offering climbing structures, hiding spots, and interactive toys, stimulate their natural behaviors and prevent boredom. Regular handling and social interaction also contribute to their overall well-being, as long as it is done gently and respectfully.

In conclusion, maintaining the health and wellness of your bearded dragon requires a proactive approach, combining preventive care, proper nutrition, and regular veterinary visits. By understanding common health issues, recognizing signs of illness, and implementing effective care strategies, you can ensure your bearded dragon leads a happy, healthy life. Remember, the key to successful bearded dragon ownership lies in your commitment to providing the best possible care, creating a thriving environment, and staying informed about their unique needs. With dedication and knowledge, you can enjoy a rewarding and fulfilling relationship with your bearded dragon, watching them flourish under your attentive care.

4.1 Identifying common health issues

Identifying common health issues in bearded dragons is a critical aspect of ensuring their well-being and longevity. As a responsible pet owner, understanding these health problems and their early symptoms can make a significant difference in the quality of life for your scaly companion. One of the most prevalent health issues in bearded dragons is metabolic bone disease (MBD), a condition resulting from calcium deficiency or an imbalance between calcium, phosphorus, and vitamin D3. MBD can lead to weakened bones, deformities, and even fractures. Early signs include lethargy, tremors, swollen limbs, and a soft or rubbery jaw. In severe cases, dragons may exhibit difficulty in moving or climbing. Preventing MBD involves ensuring a diet rich in calcium, proper UVB lighting to facilitate vitamin D3 synthesis, and maintaining a balanced ratio of calcium to phosphorus in their diet. Respiratory infections are another common ailment in bearded dragons, often caused by inadequate temperature gradients or high humidity levels in their enclosure. Symptoms include wheezing, mucus discharge from the nose or mouth, labored breathing, and lethargy. Early detection and treatment are crucial, as untreated respiratory infections can lead to pneumonia and other severe complications. Maintaining optimal temperature and humidity levels, along with regular cleaning of the habitat, can help prevent these infections. Impaction, a condition where a bearded dragon's digestive tract becomes blocked, is often caused by ingesting substrate materials, large food items, or indigestible objects. Symptoms of impaction include lack of appetite, lethargy, bloating, and difficulty in defecating. To prevent impaction, it's essential to provide a suitable substrate, such as reptile carpet or paper towels, and ensure that food items are appropriately sized. In some cases, gentle massages and warm baths can help alleviate mild impactions, but severe cases may require veterinary intervention. Parasites, both internal and external, are another health concern for bearded dragons. Internal parasites, such as pinworms and coccidia, can cause weight loss, diarrhea, and a general decline in health. Regular fecal examinations by a veterinarian can help detect and treat these parasites early. External parasites, like mites and ticks, can cause skin irritation, anemia, and stress. Regularly inspecting your bearded dragon and their habitat for signs of parasites, along with maintaining a clean environment, can help prevent infestations. Additionally, bearded dragons are prone to a variety of skin conditions, including fungal infections and scale rot. Fungal infections often present as discolored, crusty, or flaky patches on the skin, while scale rot can cause ulcers and open sores. Both conditions require prompt veterinary care and can be prevented by maintaining proper humidity levels and ensuring a clean habitat. Another common health issue is dehydration, which can lead to kidney problems and other complications. Signs of dehydration include sunken eyes, wrinkled skin, and lethargy.

Providing a shallow water dish, misting the enclosure, and offering water-rich foods can help keep your bearded dragon hydrated. In some cases, dehydration may require veterinary intervention with subcutaneous fluids. Bearded dragons can also suffer from nutritional deficiencies, which can manifest as poor growth, lethargy, and weakened immune function. A varied diet that includes a mix of insects, vegetables, and occasional fruits, along with appropriate supplementation, can help prevent these deficiencies. Regularly monitoring your bearded dragon's weight and overall condition can provide early indicators of nutritional issues. In addition to these common health problems, bearded dragons may also experience stress-related illnesses. Stress can be caused by a variety of factors, including improper handling, inadequate habitat conditions, and changes in their environment. Signs of stress include darkening of the beard, loss of appetite, and increased hiding behavior. Providing a stable and enriched environment, along with gentle handling, can help reduce stress levels. Lastly, bearded dragons are susceptible to a range of other health issues, including liver disease, kidney disease, and reproductive problems. Regular veterinary check-ups, a balanced diet, and proper habitat conditions are essential in preventing and managing these conditions. Understanding and identifying common health issues in bearded dragons is a crucial part of responsible pet ownership. By being vigilant and proactive, you can ensure that your bearded dragon remains healthy and happy for years to come.

4.2 Preventive care strategies

Preventive care strategies for bearded dragons are essential to ensure these captivating reptiles lead healthy, fulfilling lives. One of the most critical aspects of preventive care is providing proper lighting. Bearded dragons require a specific spectrum of UVB light to synthesize vitamin D3, which is crucial for calcium absorption. Without adequate UVB exposure, bearded dragons can develop metabolic bone disease (MBD), a debilitating condition that weakens their bones. To prevent this, it's vital to invest in a high-quality UVB bulb and replace it every six months, as the UVB output diminishes over time. Position the bulb within 12-18 inches of the basking spot and ensure there are no obstructions, such as glass or plastic, that could filter out the beneficial rays. Additionally, providing a gradient of temperatures within the enclosure is crucial. Bearded dragons thrive in a habitat with a basking spot temperature of 95-110°F and a cooler area around 75-85°F. This temperature gradient allows them to thermoregulate, moving between warmer and cooler areas to maintain their optimal body temperature. Using a combination of heat lamps and ceramic heat emitters can help achieve this gradient. Monitoring temperatures with reliable thermometers placed at both the basking spot and the cooler end of the enclosure is essential to ensure consistency.

Diet is another cornerstone of preventive care. Bearded dragons are omnivores, requiring a balanced diet of insects and vegetables. Juveniles need a higher protein intake, primarily from insects like crickets, dubia roaches, and mealworms, while adults should have a diet consisting of 80% vegetables and 20% insects. Leafy greens such as collard greens, mustard greens, and dandelion greens are excellent choices, while fruits should be offered sparingly due to their high sugar content. It's also important to gut-load insects with nutritious foods before feeding them to your bearded dragon, ensuring they receive the maximum nutritional benefit. Dusting insects with calcium powder three to four times a week and a multivitamin supplement once a week can help prevent deficiencies. Hydration is often overlooked but is equally vital. Bearded dragons may not drink from standing water, so misting their vegetables and providing a shallow water dish can encourage hydration. Additionally, offering a bath once a week can help with hydration and aid in shedding.

Habitat maintenance plays a significant role in preventive care. Regular cleaning of the enclosure is necessary to prevent the buildup of harmful bacteria and parasites. Spot clean daily to remove feces and uneaten food, and perform a thorough cleaning of the entire enclosure, including the substrate, hides, and decor, at least once a month. Using a reptile-safe disinfectant ensures that harmful pathogens are eliminated without posing a risk to your bearded dragon. Substrate choice is also crucial; avoid loose substrates like sand or wood chips, which can cause impaction if ingested. Instead, opt for reptile carpet, paper towels, or tile, which are easier to clean and pose less risk.

Behavioral observation is a key preventive measure. Bearded dragons are creatures of habit, and any deviation from their normal behavior can be an early indicator of health issues. Regularly observing your bearded dragon's eating habits, activity levels, and general demeanor can help you catch potential problems early. For example, a sudden loss of appetite, lethargy, or changes in stool consistency can signal underlying health issues that require prompt attention. Stress is another factor that can impact a bearded dragon's health. Ensuring a stable and enriching environment with plenty of hiding spots and opportunities for exploration can reduce stress levels. Avoid handling your bearded dragon excessively, especially during shedding or when they are adjusting to a new environment, as this can also contribute to stress.

Preventive care also extends to regular health checks. While bearded dragons are generally hardy reptiles, they can still fall prey to various health issues. Scheduling annual check-ups with a reptile veterinarian can help catch potential problems early. During these visits, the vet can perform a thorough examination, including checking for parasites, assessing weight and body condition, and providing guidance on any necessary dietary or environmental adjustments. Additionally, keeping a health log for your bearded dragon can be beneficial. Recording their weight, shedding cycles, and any notable changes in behavior or appearance can help you and your vet track their health over time.

Incorporating enrichment activities into your bearded dragon's routine is another preventive care strategy. Providing opportunities for mental and physical stimulation can enhance their overall well-being. This can include offering a variety of climbing structures, interactive toys, and opportunities for supervised exploration outside of their enclosure. Enrichment activities not only keep your bearded dragon engaged but also promote natural behaviors, such as hunting and foraging, which can contribute to their physical health.

Finally, educating yourself continuously about bearded dragon care is an ongoing preventive measure. The more knowledgeable you are, the better equipped you'll be to provide optimal care for your bearded dragon. Joining online forums, attending reptile expos, and reading reputable sources can keep you updated on the latest care techniques and potential health risks. By staying informed and proactive, you can ensure that your bearded dragon enjoys a long, healthy, and happy life.

In conclusion, preventive care for bearded dragons encompasses a holistic approach that includes proper lighting, a balanced diet, habitat maintenance, behavioral observation, regular health checks, enrichment activities, and continuous education. By implementing these strategies, you can create a thriving environment for your bearded dragon, minimizing the risk of health issues and enhancing their quality of life.

4.3 Nutrition and its impact on health

Nutrition plays a pivotal role in the overall health and well-being of bearded dragons, and understanding the intricacies of their dietary needs is essential for any responsible owner. Bearded dragons, native to the arid regions of Australia, have evolved to thrive on a diet that mimics their natural environment. This includes a balanced intake of proteins, vegetables, and occasional fruits. A well-rounded diet ensures that these reptiles receive the necessary vitamins, minerals, and nutrients to support their growth, immune system, and overall vitality. One of the most critical aspects of bearded dragon nutrition is the balance between calcium and phosphorus. Calcium is vital for bone health, muscle function, and metabolic processes. A deficiency in calcium can lead to metabolic bone disease (MBD), a common and often debilitating condition in bearded dragons. MBD can cause weakened bones, fractures, and severe deformities. To prevent this, it is crucial to provide a diet rich in calcium and to supplement with calcium powder, especially for young and growing dragons. Phosphorus, on the other hand, should be carefully monitored, as an excess can interfere with calcium absorption. The ideal calcium-to-phosphorus ratio in a bearded dragon's diet is 2:1. This balance can be achieved by offering a variety of leafy greens such as collard greens, mustard greens, and dandelion greens, which are high in calcium and low in phosphorus. Protein is another essential component of a bearded dragon's diet, particularly for juveniles who require more protein to support their rapid growth. Insects such as crickets, mealworms, and dubia roaches are excellent sources of protein. However, it is important to gut-load these insects with nutritious foods before feeding them to your dragon, ensuring they provide maximum nutritional value. Additionally, dusting insects with a calcium supplement before feeding can help maintain the necessary calcium levels. As bearded dragons mature, their protein needs decrease, and their diet should shift towards a higher proportion of vegetables. Adult bearded dragons typically thrive on a diet consisting of 70-80% vegetables and 20-30% protein. This transition helps prevent obesity and related health issues, which can be common in captive dragons. Vegetables should be varied and include a mix of leafy greens, squash, bell peppers, and carrots. Occasional fruits can be offered as treats, but they should not make up a significant portion of the diet due to their high sugar content. Hydration is another critical aspect of nutrition that is often overlooked. Bearded dragons obtain moisture from their food and by drinking water. Providing a shallow water dish in their enclosure is essential, but it is also important to mist their vegetables lightly to ensure they stay hydrated. Dehydration can lead to kidney problems and other health issues, so monitoring their water intake is crucial. Nutritional deficiencies can have severe consequences for bearded dragons. For example, a lack of vitamin A can lead to respiratory infections, eye problems, and poor skin health. To prevent this, it is important to include vitamin A-rich foods such as carrots, sweet potatoes, and butternut squash in their diet. However, care must be taken not to over-supplement, as excessive vitamin A can be toxic. Another common deficiency is vitamin D3, which is essential for calcium absorption. In the wild, bearded dragons obtain vitamin D3 through exposure to natural sunlight. In captivity, providing UVB lighting in their enclosure is critical to ensure they synthesize vitamin D3 effectively. Without adequate UVB lighting, even a diet rich in calcium will not prevent metabolic bone disease. Case studies have shown the dramatic impact of proper nutrition on bearded dragon health. For instance, a study conducted by the University of Queensland found that bearded dragons fed a balanced diet with appropriate supplementation had significantly lower incidences of metabolic bone disease and other health issues compared to those with imbalanced diets. Another case involved a bearded dragon named Spike, who was rescued in a malnourished state with severe MBD. Through a carefully managed diet rich in calcium, vitamin D3, and other essential nutrients, Spike's condition improved dramatically, showcasing the power of proper nutrition in recovery and health maintenance. In conclusion, understanding and implementing a balanced diet is fundamental to the health and longevity of bearded dragons. By providing a variety of nutrient-rich foods, ensuring proper supplementation, and maintaining hydration, owners can prevent common health issues and support their bearded dragon's overall well-being. The impact of nutrition on health cannot be overstated, and with the right knowledge and care, bearded dragons can thrive and lead healthy, vibrant lives.

4.4 Recognizing signs of stress and illness

Recognizing signs of stress and illness in bearded dragons is crucial for ensuring their well-being and longevity. As a responsible owner, it's essential to be vigilant and observant, as these reptiles often exhibit subtle cues that indicate their health status. Stress and illness can manifest in various ways, and understanding these signs can help you take timely action to prevent further complications.

One of the most common indicators of stress in bearded dragons is a change in behavior. A normally active and curious dragon may become lethargic, spending more time hiding or basking in one spot. This sudden shift in activity levels can be a red flag, signaling that something is amiss. Additionally, a stressed bearded dragon might exhibit a loss of appetite. If your dragon is consistently refusing food or showing disinterest in their favorite treats, it could be a sign of underlying stress or illness. It's important to monitor their eating habits closely, as prolonged periods of anorexia can lead to severe health issues.

Physical signs of stress and illness are also critical to recognize. One of the most noticeable symptoms is weight loss. Regularly weighing your bearded dragon can help you track any significant changes in their weight. A healthy dragon should maintain a consistent weight, and any sudden loss should be investigated promptly. Another physical sign to watch for is changes in skin color. Bearded dragons can change color for various reasons, including temperature regulation and mood. However, if you notice persistent darkening or unusual color patterns, it could indicate stress or illness. For instance, a darkened beard, even when the dragon is not displaying aggressive behavior, can be a sign of discomfort or health issues.

Shedding problems are another indicator of potential stress or illness. While shedding is a natural process for bearded dragons, difficulties in shedding can point to underlying health problems. Retained shed, where patches of old skin remain stuck to the body, can cause discomfort and lead to infections if not addressed. Ensuring proper humidity levels and providing shedding aids, such as rough surfaces or shedding sprays, can help alleviate this issue.

Respiratory issues are a serious concern and can often be identified through specific symptoms. Wheezing, labored breathing, or mucus around the nostrils and mouth are clear signs of respiratory distress. These symptoms can be caused by bacterial or viral infections, often exacerbated by improper habitat conditions, such as inadequate temperature or humidity levels. Immediate veterinary attention is required to diagnose and treat respiratory infections effectively.

Another critical aspect of recognizing stress and illness is observing changes in fecal matter. Healthy bearded dragon feces should be well-formed and consistent in appearance. Diarrhea, constipation, or the presence of undigested food can indicate gastrointestinal issues or parasitic infections. Regular fecal examinations by a veterinarian can help detect and treat these problems early.

Behavioral changes, such as increased aggression or unusual docility, can also be indicative of stress or illness. A typically docile dragon that suddenly becomes aggressive or a normally active dragon that becomes unusually calm should be closely monitored. These behavioral shifts can be responses to pain, discomfort, or environmental stressors. Identifying and addressing the root cause of these changes is essential for restoring your dragon's well-being.

Case studies have shown that environmental factors play a significant role in the health of bearded dragons. For example, a study conducted on a group of bearded dragons revealed that those kept in enclosures with inadequate temperature gradients and poor lighting exhibited higher levels of stress and were more prone to illnesses. Ensuring that your dragon's habitat mimics their natural environment, with appropriate temperature zones, UVB lighting, and hiding spots, can significantly reduce stress levels and promote overall health.

Another case study highlighted the impact of diet on the health of bearded dragons. Dragons fed a balanced diet, rich in essential nutrients and appropriately supplemented with vitamins and minerals, showed fewer signs of stress and illness compared to those with imbalanced diets. Providing a varied diet that includes a mix of insects, leafy greens, and occasional fruits can help maintain your dragon's health and prevent nutritional deficiencies.

In addition to environmental and dietary factors, social interactions can influence the stress levels of bearded dragons. While they are generally solitary creatures, some dragons may become stressed if housed with other dragons, especially if there is competition for resources or dominance disputes. Observing your dragon's interactions and ensuring they have a peaceful and solitary environment can help reduce stress.

Preventive care strategies, such as regular health check-ups and maintaining optimal habitat conditions, are crucial for minimizing the risk of stress and illness. Regular veterinary visits can help detect potential health issues early and provide guidance on proper care practices. Additionally, maintaining a clean and hygienic enclosure, with regular substrate changes and disinfection, can prevent the buildup of harmful bacteria and parasites.

In conclusion, recognizing signs of stress and illness in bearded dragons requires a keen eye and a proactive approach. By closely monitoring their behavior, physical condition, and environmental factors, you can ensure timely intervention and provide the best possible care for your scaly companion. Understanding the subtle cues and taking preventive measures can significantly enhance your dragon's quality of life and ensure they thrive in their home environment.

4.5 When to seek veterinary care

When it comes to bearded dragon care, understanding when to seek veterinary care is crucial for ensuring the health and well-being of your scaly companion. While bearded dragons are generally hardy reptiles, they can still experience a range of health issues that require professional attention. Knowing the signs of severe symptoms and emergencies can make a significant difference in the outcome of your pet's health. One of the most common scenarios that necessitate a visit to the vet is when your bearded dragon exhibits signs of respiratory infections. These infections can manifest through symptoms such as wheezing, labored breathing, excessive mucus around the nostrils and mouth, and a noticeable decrease in activity levels. Respiratory infections can quickly escalate if left untreated, leading to more severe complications. Therefore, it is imperative to seek veterinary care at the first sign of respiratory distress.

Another critical situation that warrants immediate veterinary attention is when your bearded dragon shows signs of impaction. Impaction occurs when a blockage forms in the digestive tract, often due to the ingestion of substrate, large food items, or indigestible materials. Symptoms of impaction include a lack of bowel movements, a distended abdomen, lethargy, and a refusal to eat. If you suspect your bearded dragon is impacted, do not attempt to treat it at home. A veterinarian can perform diagnostic tests, such as X-rays, to determine the severity of the impaction and provide appropriate treatment, which may include laxatives, enemas, or even surgery in severe cases.

Metabolic bone disease (MBD) is another condition that requires veterinary intervention. MBD is caused by a deficiency in calcium or vitamin D3, leading to weakened bones, deformities, and fractures. Signs of MBD include tremors, difficulty moving, swollen limbs, and a soft jaw. Early detection and treatment are crucial to prevent irreversible damage. A veterinarian can prescribe calcium supplements, UVB lighting adjustments, and dietary changes to manage and treat MBD effectively.

Parasite infestations, both internal and external, are also common in bearded dragons and necessitate veterinary care. Internal parasites, such as worms and protozoa, can cause symptoms like weight loss, diarrhea, and a bloated abdomen. External parasites, such as mites, can lead to excessive scratching, shedding issues, and visible tiny black or red dots on the skin. A veterinarian can perform fecal tests to identify internal parasites and provide deworming medications. For external parasites, they can recommend appropriate treatments and cleaning protocols to eradicate the infestation.

Injuries, whether from falls, bites, or other accidents, also require veterinary attention. Bearded dragons are prone to injuries due to their active nature and curiosity. If your bearded dragon sustains a cut, fracture, or any other injury, it is essential to seek veterinary care to prevent infection and ensure proper healing. A veterinarian can clean and dress wounds, set fractures, and provide pain management to aid in recovery.

Additionally, bearded dragons can suffer from egg-binding, a condition where a female is unable to lay her eggs. This can be life-threatening if not addressed promptly. Signs of egg-binding include a swollen abdomen, straining without producing eggs, lethargy, and loss of appetite. A veterinarian can perform diagnostic imaging to confirm egg-binding and may need to administer medications to induce egg-laying or perform surgery to remove the eggs.

Another scenario that requires immediate veterinary care is when your bearded dragon exhibits signs of severe dehydration. Dehydration can occur due to inadequate water intake, high temperatures, or underlying health issues. Symptoms include sunken eyes, wrinkled skin, lethargy, and a lack of appetite. A veterinarian can provide fluids through injections or oral rehydration solutions to restore hydration levels and address any underlying causes.

Moreover, bearded dragons can experience neurological issues, such as seizures or head tilting, which can indicate underlying health problems like infections, trauma, or metabolic imbalances. If your bearded dragon exhibits any neurological symptoms, it is crucial to seek veterinary care immediately. A veterinarian can perform diagnostic tests, such as blood work or imaging, to determine the cause and provide appropriate treatment.

In some cases, bearded dragons may develop tumors or other growths that require veterinary evaluation. While not all growths are malignant, it is essential to have them examined by a veterinarian to determine their nature and decide on the best course of action. Treatment options may include surgical removal, biopsy, or monitoring for any changes.

Behavioral changes can also signal the need for veterinary care. If your bearded dragon suddenly becomes aggressive, lethargic, or exhibits unusual behaviors, it may be a sign of an underlying health issue. A veterinarian can conduct a thorough examination to identify any potential problems and provide guidance on addressing them.

Lastly, it is essential to seek veterinary care for routine check-ups and preventive care. Regular veterinary visits can help detect potential health issues early, ensuring timely intervention and treatment. During these visits, a veterinarian can perform physical exams, fecal tests, and blood work to monitor your bearded dragon's health and provide recommendations for diet, lighting, and habitat adjustments.

In conclusion, knowing when to seek veterinary care for your bearded dragon is vital for maintaining their health and well-being. Respiratory infections, impaction, metabolic bone disease, parasite infestations, injuries, egg-binding, dehydration, neurological issues, tumors, and behavioral changes are all scenarios that require professional veterinary attention. By recognizing the signs of these conditions and seeking timely veterinary care, you can ensure that your bearded dragon receives the best possible care and enjoys a long, healthy life.

4.6 Creating a wellness routine

Creating a wellness routine for your bearded dragon is an essential aspect of ensuring their long-term health and happiness. This routine should be comprehensive, covering various aspects of care, including regular health check-ups, habitat cleaning, and consistent monitoring of your bearded dragon's behavior and physical condition. Establishing a wellness routine not only helps in early detection of potential health issues but also fosters a strong bond between you and your pet, as they become accustomed to the care and attention you provide.

To begin with, regular health check-ups are crucial. These should be conducted both at home and with a qualified reptile veterinarian. At home, you should perform a weekly physical examination of your bearded dragon. This involves checking their eyes, nose, mouth, and skin for any signs of infection or abnormalities. Look for clear, bright eyes, a clean nose without discharge, and a healthy mouth with no signs of swelling or discoloration. The skin should be smooth and free of cuts, sores, or unusual lumps. Additionally, monitor their weight regularly using a small digital scale. Significant weight loss or gain can be an early indicator of health issues.

Scheduling annual veterinary visits is also important. A reptile vet can perform more thorough examinations, including blood tests and fecal exams, to detect parasites or other internal issues that may not be visible during a home check-up. These visits are also an opportunity to discuss any concerns you may have and to get professional advice on your bearded dragon's care.

Cleaning your bearded dragon's habitat is another critical component of a wellness routine. A clean environment reduces the risk of infections and promotes overall well-being. Daily spot cleaning involves removing uneaten food, feces, and any soiled substrate. This prevents the buildup of bacteria and keeps the habitat hygienic. Once a week, conduct a more thorough cleaning. This includes replacing the substrate, cleaning the tank walls, and disinfecting all accessories such as water bowls, hides, and decor items. Use reptile-safe cleaning products to avoid any harmful residues that could affect your bearded dragon's health.

Monitoring your bearded dragon's behavior is equally important. Bearded dragons are creatures of habit, and any significant changes in their behavior can be a sign of stress or illness. Observe their eating habits, activity levels, and social interactions. A healthy bearded dragon should have a good appetite, be active during the day, and exhibit normal social behaviors such as basking, exploring, and interacting with you. If you notice a decrease in appetite, lethargy, or unusual aggression, it may be time to investigate further or consult a vet.

Incorporating enrichment activities into your bearded dragon's routine is beneficial for their mental and physical health. These activities can include providing new items for them to explore, such as different types of hides, branches, and rocks. You can also introduce foraging activities by hiding food around their enclosure, encouraging them to use their natural hunting instincts. Regular handling and interaction with your bearded dragon also contribute to their well-being. Gentle handling helps them become accustomed to human contact, reducing stress during routine care and vet visits.

Hydration is another key aspect of a wellness routine. Ensure your bearded dragon has access to fresh water at all times. Some bearded dragons may not drink from a bowl, so misting their enclosure or providing a shallow water dish for them to soak in can help maintain proper hydration. Bathing your bearded dragon once a week in lukewarm water can also aid in hydration and help with shedding.

Diet plays a significant role in your bearded dragon's health. A balanced diet consisting of appropriate vegetables, fruits, and live insects is essential. Regularly review and adjust their diet based on their age, size, and health status. Young bearded dragons require more protein, while adults need a diet higher in vegetables. Supplementing their diet with calcium and vitamin D3 is crucial to prevent metabolic bone disease, a common issue in captive reptiles.

Finally, maintaining proper temperature and lighting in your bearded dragon's habitat is vital for their health. Ensure that the basking area is at the correct temperature, typically between 95-110°F, and that there is a cooler area in the tank for them to regulate their body temperature. UVB lighting is essential for calcium metabolism and overall health. Replace UVB bulbs every six months, as their effectiveness diminishes over time.

In conclusion, creating a wellness routine for your bearded dragon involves a combination of regular health check-ups, habitat cleaning, behavior monitoring, enrichment activities, proper hydration, a balanced diet, and maintaining appropriate temperature and lighting. By establishing and adhering to this routine, you can ensure that your bearded dragon remains healthy, happy, and well-cared for. This routine not only benefits your pet but also enhances your experience as a responsible and knowledgeable bearded dragon owner.

5. Understanding bearded dragon behavior

Understanding bearded dragon behavior is a fascinating and essential aspect of ensuring the well-being and happiness of these unique reptiles. Bearded dragons, native to the arid regions of Australia, exhibit a wide range of behaviors that can be both intriguing and perplexing to their owners. By delving into their natural behaviors and social interactions, owners can better interpret their pets' actions and needs, fostering a deeper bond and providing a more enriching environment for their scaly companions.

One of the most distinctive behaviors of bearded dragons is their body language, which serves as a primary mode of communication. Bearded dragons use a variety of physical cues to express their emotions and intentions. For instance, head bobbing is a common behavior observed in both males and females. Rapid head bobbing is often a sign of dominance or aggression, particularly during territorial disputes or mating rituals. Conversely, slow head bobbing can indicate submission or acknowledgment of another dragon's presence. Understanding these nuances can help owners gauge their dragon's mood and respond appropriately.

Another notable behavior is the bearded dragon's ability to puff out its beard, which is a display of dominance or defense. When threatened or agitated, a bearded dragon will darken and expand its beard, making itself appear larger and more intimidating. This behavior is often accompanied by an open mouth and hissing sound, further emphasizing the dragon's discomfort or aggression. Recognizing this behavior is crucial for owners, as it signals that the dragon is feeling threatened and may need space or a change in its environment to feel secure.

Bearded dragons are also known for their unique arm-waving behavior, which is typically a sign of submission or recognition. This slow, circular motion of one front leg is often seen in younger dragons or females, indicating that they are not a threat. In social settings, arm-waving can help establish a hierarchy among dragons, reducing the likelihood of aggressive encounters. For owners, witnessing this behavior can provide insight into their dragon's social dynamics and overall comfort level.

In addition to body language, vocalizations and sounds play a role in bearded dragon communication, although they are generally less vocal than other pets. Hissing is the most common sound, usually indicating fear or aggression. It is essential for owners to recognize this sound and understand its context, as it often precedes defensive behaviors like beard puffing. By identifying the source of their dragon's distress, owners can take steps to alleviate it and create a more comfortable environment.

Territorial behaviors are another critical aspect of bearded dragon behavior. In the wild, bearded dragons establish and defend territories to secure resources such as food, basking spots, and mates. In captivity, this instinct can manifest as aggression towards other dragons or even their reflections. Owners should be mindful of their dragon's territorial nature and provide ample space and hiding spots to reduce stress and prevent conflicts. Introducing new dragons to an established habitat should be done gradually and under close supervision to ensure a smooth transition.

Social interactions with humans are an integral part of bearded dragon behavior, as these reptiles can form bonds with their owners. Regular handling and gentle interactions can help build trust and reduce stress. Bearded dragons often enjoy being held and may even seek out human contact. However, it is essential to approach handling with care, as improper techniques can lead to stress or injury. Owners should support their dragon's body fully and avoid sudden movements that could startle them. Over time, consistent and positive interactions can strengthen the bond between dragon and owner, leading to a more fulfilling relationship.

Recognizing signs of stress is crucial for maintaining a bearded dragon's health and well-being. Stress can manifest in various ways, including changes in appetite, lethargy, or unusual behaviors such as glass surfing (repeatedly running along the sides of the enclosure). Identifying the root cause of stress, whether it be environmental factors, health issues, or social dynamics, is essential for addressing it effectively. Providing a stable and enriching environment, with appropriate temperature, lighting, and hiding spots, can help mitigate stress and promote a sense of security.

Play and stimulation are vital components of a bearded dragon's daily routine. These reptiles are naturally curious and benefit from activities that engage their minds and bodies. Owners can introduce a variety of toys and enrichment items, such as climbing structures, tunnels, and interactive feeders, to keep their dragons entertained. Supervised exploration outside the enclosure, in a safe and controlled environment, can also provide mental and physical stimulation. Encouraging natural behaviors, such as hunting for live insects, can further enhance their quality of life.

Understanding bearded dragon behavior requires a holistic approach, considering both their natural instincts and individual personalities. Each dragon is unique, and owners should take the time to observe and learn their pet's specific behaviors and preferences. By fostering a deep understanding of their dragon's actions and needs, owners can create a harmonious and enriching environment that promotes the well-being and happiness of their scaly companion. This journey of discovery not only strengthens the bond between dragon and owner but also enhances the overall experience of bearded dragon ownership, making it a truly rewarding adventure.

5.1 Body language basics

Understanding the body language of bearded dragons is crucial for any owner aiming to provide the best care for their scaly companion. These reptiles, native to the arid regions of Australia, communicate a wealth of information through their body language, which can reveal their mood, health, and overall well-being. By paying close attention to their posture, tail positioning, and eye movements, owners can gain valuable insights into their pet's needs and emotions, ensuring a happy and healthy life for their bearded dragon.

One of the most fundamental aspects of bearded dragon body language is their posture. When a bearded dragon is relaxed and content, it will often lie flat on its belly with its limbs splayed out to the sides. This position indicates that the dragon feels safe and comfortable in its environment. Conversely, a bearded dragon that is feeling threatened or stressed may puff up its body, flatten itself against the ground, and open its mouth wide in a display known as "gaping." This behavior is a defensive mechanism designed to make the dragon appear larger and more intimidating to potential predators. Owners should be mindful of these signals and take steps to alleviate any sources of stress in their pet's environment.

Tail positioning is another key indicator of a bearded dragon's mood. A relaxed and happy bearded dragon will typically have its tail resting gently on the ground or slightly curled around its body. In contrast, a bearded dragon that is feeling agitated or threatened may raise its tail and hold it rigidly in the air. This behavior is often accompanied by other signs of distress, such as darkening of the beard and rapid head bobbing. By observing these cues, owners can take proactive measures to calm their pet and remove any potential stressors.

Eye movements also play a significant role in bearded dragon communication. A bearded dragon that is feeling curious or alert will often have its eyes wide open and focused on its surroundings. This is a sign that the dragon is engaged and interested in its environment. On the other hand, a bearded dragon that is feeling sleepy or unwell may have its eyes partially closed or even shut completely. This can be an indication that the dragon is not feeling its best and may require closer monitoring or a visit to the veterinarian. Additionally, bearded dragons may engage in a behavior known as "eye bulging," where they temporarily bulge their eyes out of their sockets. This can be alarming to new owners, but it is usually a normal behavior associated with shedding or eye cleaning.

To further illustrate the importance of understanding bearded dragon body language, consider the case of a bearded dragon named Spike. Spike's owner, Alex, noticed that Spike had been spending more time hiding and appeared to be less active than usual. By closely observing Spike's body language, Alex noticed that Spike's tail was often held high and rigid, and his beard had darkened significantly. Recognizing these signs of stress, Alex made several changes to Spike's habitat, including adjusting the temperature and adding more hiding spots. Within a few days, Spike's behavior improved, and he returned to his usual, active self. This example highlights how attentive observation and prompt action can significantly impact a bearded dragon's well-being.

Research has also shown that bearded dragons use body language to communicate with each other. In a study conducted by the University of Melbourne, researchers observed interactions between wild bearded dragons and noted several distinct behaviors used for social communication. For example, head bobbing is a common behavior used by male bearded dragons to assert dominance and establish territory. A rapid series of head bobs is often a sign of aggression, while slower, more deliberate head bobs can indicate a more submissive or friendly intent. Additionally, arm waving is a behavior commonly observed in female bearded dragons and juveniles. This slow, circular motion of one front limb is a sign of submission and is often used to signal to other dragons that they pose no threat.

Understanding these social behaviors can also help owners interpret their pet's interactions with other bearded dragons or even with humans. For instance, if a bearded dragon begins head bobbing rapidly when approached by its owner, it may be feeling threatened or territorial. In such cases, it is important for the owner to approach slowly and calmly, allowing the dragon to become accustomed to their presence. Conversely, if a bearded dragon engages in arm waving when approached, it is likely signaling submission and may be more receptive to handling.

In addition to these specific behaviors, bearded dragons also use a variety of other body language cues to communicate their needs and emotions. For example, a bearded dragon that is feeling cold may flatten its body and spread out its limbs to maximize surface area and absorb more heat from its surroundings. This behavior, known as "pancaking," is a clear indication that the dragon requires more warmth. On the other hand, a bearded dragon that is feeling too hot may gape its mouth open and hold its body away from the heat source. This behavior helps the dragon regulate its body temperature and cool down.

Another important aspect of bearded dragon body language is their use of color changes. Bearded dragons have the ability to change the color of their skin to some extent, and these changes can provide valuable information about their mood and health. For example, a bearded dragon that is feeling stressed or threatened may darken its beard and body, making itself appear more intimidating. Conversely, a bearded dragon that is feeling relaxed and content may display brighter, more vibrant colors. Owners should pay close attention to these color changes and consider them in conjunction with other body language cues to gain a comprehensive understanding of their pet's emotional state.

In conclusion, understanding the body language of bearded dragons is essential for providing the best care and ensuring the well-being of these fascinating reptiles. By closely observing their posture, tail positioning, eye movements, and color changes, owners can gain valuable insights into their pet's mood, health, and overall needs. This knowledge allows owners to create a more enriching and supportive environment for their bearded dragon, ultimately leading to a happier and healthier pet. Whether you are a first-time owner like Alex or a seasoned reptile enthusiast, taking the time to learn and interpret your bearded dragon's body language will undoubtedly enhance your experience and strengthen the bond with your scaly companion.

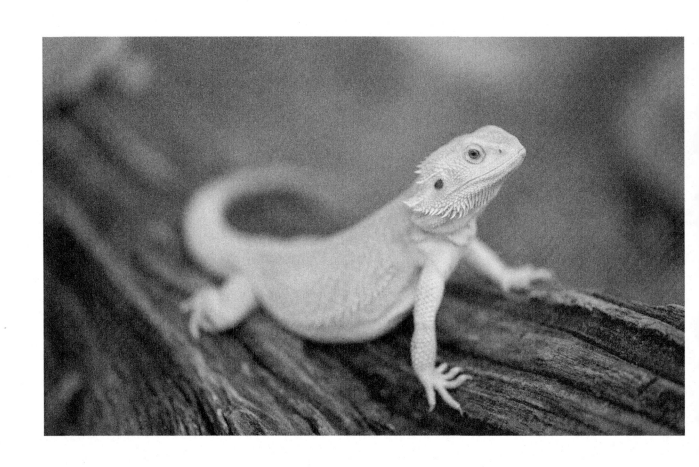

5.2 Vocalizations and sounds

Bearded dragons, though often perceived as silent creatures, actually possess a range of vocalizations and sounds that convey various messages and emotions. Understanding these vocal cues is crucial for any bearded dragon owner, as it allows for better communication and a deeper bond with their scaly companion. One of the most common sounds a bearded dragon makes is hissing. This sound is typically a sign of distress or discomfort and can be triggered by various factors such as feeling threatened, being handled improperly, or encountering a new and unfamiliar environment. For instance, if Alex, our 28-year-old tech professional, notices their bearded dragon hissing when introduced to a new habitat setup, it might indicate that the dragon is feeling overwhelmed or insecure. In such cases, it's essential to give the dragon time to acclimate and ensure that the environment is as stress-free as possible.

Another sound that bearded dragons make is clicking. This noise can be a bit more ambiguous, as it might signify different things depending on the context. Clicking can sometimes be heard when a bearded dragon is eating, especially if they are consuming harder food items like insects with exoskeletons. However, if the clicking is frequent and not associated with feeding, it could indicate a respiratory issue. Respiratory infections are not uncommon in bearded dragons and can be caused by improper humidity levels or a dirty habitat. If Alex hears persistent clicking, it would be wise to consult a veterinarian to rule out any health concerns.

Bearded dragons also produce a low, rumbling sound, somewhat akin to a growl. This sound is less common but can occur during moments of extreme agitation or when the dragon is trying to assert dominance. For example, if Alex's bearded dragon encounters another dragon or even its own reflection, it might growl to establish its territory. Understanding this sound can help Alex manage interactions between multiple dragons or prevent unnecessary stress by avoiding situations that might trigger such responses.

In addition to these sounds, bearded dragons can also make a puffing noise. This is often accompanied by the inflation of their beard, which turns black as a visual display of dominance or defense. Puffing is usually a sign that the dragon is feeling threatened or is trying to appear larger and more intimidating to ward off potential threats. If Alex notices their dragon puffing frequently, it might be necessary to evaluate the environment for stressors, such as other pets, loud noises, or sudden movements.

Interestingly, some bearded dragons have been observed making a chirping sound. This is relatively rare and not as well-documented as other vocalizations. Chirping might occur during interactions with other dragons or even during play. While the exact meaning of chirping is still a subject of study, it is generally considered a positive sound, indicating curiosity or contentment. If Alex hears their dragon chirping, it could be a sign that the dragon is happy and engaged with its surroundings.

To further illustrate the importance of understanding bearded dragon vocalizations, consider a case study involving a bearded dragon named Spike. Spike's owner, a novice reptile enthusiast, noticed that Spike would frequently hiss and puff up his beard whenever approached. Initially, the owner thought Spike was simply aggressive by nature. However, after consulting with a reptile behaviorist, it was discovered that Spike's habitat was too small and lacked adequate hiding spots, causing him to feel constantly exposed and stressed. By upgrading Spike's tank and adding more hides, the owner was able to significantly reduce Spike's stress levels, leading to fewer hissing incidents and a much calmer dragon.

Research also supports the notion that bearded dragons use vocalizations as a form of communication. A study conducted by the University of Melbourne observed that bearded dragons in captivity exhibited a range of vocal behaviors that were directly correlated with their environmental conditions and social interactions. The study found that dragons housed in enriched environments with plenty of stimulation and proper care were less likely to exhibit distress vocalizations like hissing and more likely to produce contentment sounds such as chirping.

For Alex, understanding these vocal cues can greatly enhance the care and well-being of their bearded dragon. By paying attention to the sounds their dragon makes, Alex can quickly identify when something is amiss and take appropriate action. For instance, if Alex hears hissing during handling, it might indicate that the dragon is not comfortable with the way it is being held. Adjusting the handling technique or giving the dragon more time to get used to being handled can help alleviate this issue.

Moreover, recognizing the significance of clicking sounds can prompt Alex to regularly check the humidity levels and cleanliness of the habitat, ensuring that respiratory infections are kept at bay. Similarly, understanding the context of growling or puffing can help Alex manage the dragon's interactions with other pets or its own reflection, preventing unnecessary stress and promoting a harmonious living environment.

In conclusion, the vocalizations and sounds made by bearded dragons are a vital aspect of their communication repertoire. By learning to interpret these sounds, owners like Alex can provide better care, respond appropriately to their dragon's needs, and foster a deeper, more meaningful bond with their pet. Whether it's a hiss of discomfort, a click of curiosity, or a rare chirp of contentment, each sound offers valuable insights into the dragon's emotional state and well-being. As Alex continues their journey as a bearded dragon owner, this understanding will be an indispensable tool in ensuring their scaly friend leads a happy, healthy, and enriched life.

5.3 Territorial behaviors

Territorial behaviors in bearded dragons are a fascinating and complex aspect of their natural behavior, reflecting their instincts and social interactions in the wild. Understanding these behaviors is crucial for any bearded dragon owner, as it helps in creating a harmonious environment and preventing potential conflicts. Bearded dragons are solitary creatures by nature, and their territorial instincts are deeply ingrained. In the wild, they establish and defend territories to secure resources such as food, basking spots, and mates. These behaviors are often carried over into captivity, where they may exhibit signs of aggression or dominance towards other dragons or even their own reflections.

One of the most common signs of territorial behavior in bearded dragons is head bobbing. This rapid up-and-down movement of the head is a display of dominance and is often accompanied by other aggressive behaviors such as puffing up the beard, which turns black, and flattening the body to appear larger. These displays are meant to intimidate potential rivals and assert dominance. For example, if you house two male bearded dragons in the same enclosure, you may notice them engaging in head bobbing and beard puffing as they establish their hierarchy. In some cases, this can escalate to physical confrontations, including biting and chasing, which can result in injuries.

Another territorial behavior is arm-waving, which is typically seen in submissive dragons. This slow, circular motion of the front leg is a sign of submission and is often used by females or younger dragons to signal that they are not a threat. In a captive setting, you might observe a smaller or less dominant dragon arm-waving in response to the head bobbing of a more dominant dragon. This behavior helps to reduce the likelihood of conflict by clearly communicating the dragon's submissive status.

Bearded dragons may also exhibit territorial behaviors towards their reflections. Seeing their own image in the glass of their enclosure, they may mistake it for another dragon and display aggressive behaviors such as head bobbing, beard puffing, and scratching at the glass. This can be stressful for the dragon and may lead to injuries if they persistently try to attack their reflection. To mitigate this, owners can cover the sides of the enclosure with opaque materials or rearrange the setup to minimize reflective surfaces.

Managing territorial behaviors in bearded dragons requires careful observation and intervention. One effective strategy is to provide ample space and resources within the enclosure. Ensuring that each dragon has access to its own basking spot, hiding place, and feeding area can reduce competition and the need for territorial displays. For example, in a large enclosure with multiple basking spots and hides, dragons are less likely to feel the need to defend a specific area, leading to a more peaceful coexistence.

In cases where territorial aggression becomes problematic, it may be necessary to house dragons separately. This is especially true for male bearded dragons, which are more likely to engage in aggressive behaviors towards each other. Providing individual enclosures allows each dragon to establish its own territory without the stress of competition. For instance, if you notice persistent aggression between two dragons, separating them into their own enclosures can prevent injuries and promote a healthier environment.

Research has shown that environmental enrichment can also play a role in managing territorial behaviors. Providing a stimulating environment with a variety of textures, climbing opportunities, and hiding places can keep dragons engaged and reduce the likelihood of aggressive displays. For example, adding branches, rocks, and plants to the enclosure can encourage natural behaviors such as climbing and exploring, which can help to dissipate excess energy and reduce stress.

In addition to environmental modifications, understanding the individual personalities of your bearded dragons can aid in managing territorial behaviors. Some dragons are naturally more aggressive or dominant, while others are more submissive or docile. By observing their interactions and behaviors, you can tailor your approach to meet their specific needs. For instance, a particularly dominant dragon may benefit from more space and enrichment to keep them occupied, while a more submissive dragon may require additional hiding places to feel secure.

It's also important to recognize that territorial behaviors can be influenced by factors such as age, sex, and health. Juvenile dragons are often more tolerant of each other and may exhibit fewer territorial behaviors compared to adults. However, as they mature, their territorial instincts become more pronounced. Similarly, females may display territorial behaviors during breeding season as they defend their nesting sites. Monitoring the health of your dragons is also crucial, as illness or stress can exacerbate aggressive behaviors.

Regular health checks and a balanced diet can help to maintain their overall well-being and reduce the likelihood of territorial aggression.

In conclusion, understanding and managing territorial behaviors in bearded dragons is essential for creating a harmonious and stress-free environment. By providing ample space, resources, and environmental enrichment, and by recognizing the individual personalities and needs of your dragons, you can minimize conflicts and promote a healthy, happy coexistence. Whether you're a first-time owner or an experienced reptile enthusiast, being attuned to the territorial instincts of your bearded dragons will help you to provide the best possible care and ensure their well-being.

5.4 Social interactions with humans

Understanding the social interactions between bearded dragons and their human owners is a crucial aspect of fostering a healthy and enriching relationship with these fascinating reptiles. Unlike more traditional pets like dogs or cats, bearded dragons have unique ways of expressing their emotions and building trust, which can be both rewarding and challenging for new owners. This subchapter delves into the nuances of these interactions, offering insights and practical advice to help you connect with your bearded dragon on a deeper level.

Bearded dragons, by nature, are solitary creatures in the wild, often only coming together for mating purposes. However, when kept as pets, they can develop a bond with their human caretakers, displaying behaviors that indicate trust and affection. One of the most common signs of a bearded dragon's comfort around humans is their willingness to be handled. Regular, gentle handling is essential in building this trust. Start by allowing your bearded dragon to become accustomed to your presence. Sit near their enclosure, speak softly, and let them observe you. Gradually, you can begin to offer your hand for them to explore. Patience is key; rushing this process can lead to stress and reluctance to interact.

A case study involving a bearded dragon named Spike illustrates the importance of gradual trust-building. Spike's owner, Alex, a tech professional with a keen interest in exotic pets, spent several weeks simply sitting by Spike's tank, allowing the dragon to get used to their presence. Over time, Alex began to offer small treats, like pieces of fruit, from their hand. Spike's initial wariness gave way to curiosity, and eventually, he started to climb onto Alex's hand willingly. This progression from observation to physical interaction is a testament to the effectiveness of patience and consistency in building trust.

Another critical aspect of social interaction is recognizing and responding to your bearded dragon's body language. Bearded dragons communicate a lot through their physical movements and postures. For instance, a bearded dragon that flattens its body and puffs out its beard is likely feeling threatened or stressed. Conversely, a relaxed dragon will often lie flat with its limbs spread out, basking contentedly. Understanding these cues can help you gauge your pet's comfort level and adjust your interactions accordingly. For example, if your bearded dragon displays signs of stress during handling, it might be best to give them some space and try again later.

Research has shown that bearded dragons can recognize their owners and respond to their voices and touch. A study conducted by the University of Lincoln found that bearded dragons can learn to associate their owner's presence with positive experiences, such as feeding or gentle handling. This associative learning is a powerful tool in building a strong bond with your pet. By consistently providing positive reinforcement, such as treats or gentle strokes, you can help your bearded dragon associate you with safety and comfort.

In addition to handling, interactive activities can also strengthen the bond between you and your bearded dragon. Enrichment activities, such as offering a variety of toys or creating a stimulating environment, can keep your bearded dragon engaged and mentally stimulated. For instance, some owners have found success with simple toys like small balls or climbing structures. These activities not only provide physical exercise but also encourage exploration and curiosity, which are vital for a bearded dragon's well-being.

Regular interaction and handling can also help in identifying any health issues early on. By becoming familiar with your bearded dragon's normal behavior and physical condition, you can quickly notice any changes that might indicate illness or stress. For example, a normally active and curious bearded dragon that suddenly becomes lethargic or refuses food might be experiencing health problems that require veterinary attention. This proactive approach to health monitoring is another benefit of regular social interaction.

It's also important to note that each bearded dragon has its own personality and preferences. Some may be more outgoing and eager to interact, while others might be more reserved. Respecting these individual differences is crucial in building a positive relationship. For instance, a bearded dragon that is more shy might require more time and patience to become comfortable with handling. On the other hand, a more outgoing dragon might quickly take to interactive activities and handling sessions.

The importance of creating a routine cannot be overstated. Bearded dragons thrive on consistency, and establishing a regular schedule for feeding, handling, and enrichment activities can help them feel secure and comfortable. For example, handling your bearded dragon at the same time each day can help them anticipate and become accustomed to these interactions. This routine can also help in reducing stress and anxiety, as your bearded dragon will know what to expect and when.

In conclusion, understanding and fostering social interactions with your bearded dragon is a multifaceted process that requires patience, consistency, and a keen awareness of your pet's body language and behavior. By taking the time to build trust through gentle handling, positive reinforcement, and interactive activities, you can develop a strong and rewarding bond with your bearded dragon. This bond not only enhances your pet's quality of life but also enriches your own experience as a bearded dragon owner. Whether you're a first-time owner like Alex or a seasoned reptile enthusiast, the journey of building a relationship with your bearded dragon is filled with opportunities for learning, growth, and mutual enjoyment.

5.5 Stress signals

Stress signals in bearded dragons can manifest in various ways, and understanding these signs is crucial for ensuring the well-being of your pet. One of the most common indicators of stress is glass surfing, where a bearded dragon repeatedly runs along the sides of its enclosure, often trying to climb the glass. This behavior can be caused by several factors, including a desire to escape, inadequate tank size, or a lack of environmental enrichment. For example, a case study involving a bearded dragon named Spike revealed that glass surfing ceased once the owner upgraded to a larger tank and added more hiding spots and climbing structures. Excessive hiding is another stress signal, where the dragon spends most of its time in its hideout, avoiding interaction and exposure. This can be due to environmental stressors such as improper temperature gradients, inadequate lighting, or even the presence of other pets that may be perceived as threats. Research has shown that providing a well-balanced habitat with appropriate temperature zones and UVB lighting can significantly reduce hiding behavior.

Moreover, bearded dragons may exhibit changes in their eating habits when stressed. A sudden loss of appetite or refusal to eat can be alarming for owners. For instance, a bearded dragon named Luna stopped eating for several days, causing concern for her owner, Alex. Upon closer inspection, it was discovered that the tank's temperature was too low, leading to digestive issues and stress. Once the temperature was adjusted, Luna's appetite returned to normal. Additionally, stress can cause physical changes such as darkening of the beard, which is a defensive response. This darkening is often accompanied by puffing up of the beard and body, making the dragon appear larger and more intimidating. This behavior is commonly observed when the dragon feels threatened or is exposed to new, unfamiliar environments.

Another important aspect to consider is the dragon's interaction with its owner. A normally docile bearded dragon may become aggressive or skittish when stressed. This change in behavior can be distressing for both the pet and the owner. For example, a bearded dragon named Rex, who was usually calm and friendly, started biting his owner during handling sessions. After consulting with a reptile behaviorist, it was determined that Rex was stressed due to frequent handling and lack of a proper hiding spot. Reducing the handling frequency and providing a secure hideout helped Rex return to his usual calm demeanor.

Environmental factors play a significant role in a bearded dragon's stress levels. Loud noises, sudden movements, and changes in the tank setup can all contribute to anxiety. For instance, a bearded dragon named Bella became stressed when her tank was moved to a high-traffic area of the house. She started glass surfing and refused to eat. Moving her tank back to a quieter location with less foot traffic helped alleviate her stress. It's also important to consider the social dynamics within the tank. If multiple bearded dragons are housed together, competition for resources such as food, basking spots, and hiding places can lead to stress. In one case, two bearded dragons named Max and Ruby were housed together, and Max started exhibiting signs of stress, including a darkened beard and reduced appetite. Separating the two dragons into individual tanks resolved the issue, and both dragons thrived in their new environments.

Creating a calming environment for your bearded dragon involves several key elements. First, ensure that the tank is appropriately sized and equipped with the necessary environmental enrichment, such as climbing structures, hiding spots, and basking areas. Regularly monitor the temperature and lighting to maintain optimal conditions. Additionally, minimize exposure to loud noises and sudden movements, and provide a consistent routine for feeding and handling. It's also beneficial to observe your dragon's behavior closely and make adjustments as needed. For example, if your dragon seems stressed during handling, try reducing the frequency and duration of handling sessions, and always approach your dragon calmly and gently.

In conclusion, recognizing and addressing stress signals in bearded dragons is essential for their health and well-being. By understanding the common signs of stress, such as glass surfing, excessive hiding, changes in eating habits, and physical changes, owners can take proactive steps to create a calming environment for their pets. Providing a well-balanced habitat, minimizing environmental stressors, and observing your dragon's behavior closely can help ensure that your bearded dragon remains happy and healthy.

5.6 Play and stimulation

Engaging and stimulating a bearded dragon is essential for their mental and physical well-being, and understanding the types of activities that can captivate these fascinating reptiles is crucial for any owner. Bearded dragons, with their inquisitive nature and active disposition, thrive on a variety of enriching activities that mimic their natural behaviors and environments. Providing appropriate toys and games not only keeps them entertained but also promotes their overall health and happiness. One of the most effective ways to stimulate a bearded dragon is through interactive play. Unlike traditional pets, bearded dragons may not chase a ball or fetch a stick, but they do enjoy activities that engage their hunting instincts. For instance, using a laser pointer can be an excellent way to encourage your bearded dragon to move around and exercise. The small, darting light mimics the movement of insects, prompting your dragon to chase and pounce, which is both mentally stimulating and physically beneficial. However, it is important to ensure that the laser pointer is used safely, avoiding direct contact with the dragon's eyes.

Another engaging activity involves the use of live prey. Bearded dragons are natural hunters, and offering live insects such as crickets or dubia roaches can provide both a nutritious meal and an opportunity for exercise. Setting up a small, controlled environment where the dragon can hunt these insects can be incredibly enriching. This not only satisfies their predatory instincts but also encourages natural behaviors like stalking and pouncing. Additionally, incorporating a variety of insects can prevent dietary monotony and keep your dragon interested in their meals. Beyond hunting, bearded dragons also benefit from environmental enrichment. Creating a dynamic habitat with various textures, levels, and hiding spots can stimulate their curiosity and encourage exploration. Incorporating branches, rocks, and tunnels can provide opportunities for climbing and basking, which are essential activities for their physical health. Moreover, changing the layout of their enclosure periodically can keep their environment fresh and exciting, preventing boredom.

Toys specifically designed for reptiles can also be a great addition to your bearded dragon's habitat. Items such as small balls, mirrors, and puzzle feeders can provide mental stimulation. Puzzle feeders, in particular, are excellent for encouraging problem-solving skills. These devices require the dragon to figure out how to access their food, which can be both challenging and rewarding. Mirrors can also be intriguing for bearded dragons, as they may react to their reflection, thinking it is another dragon. This can stimulate social behaviors and provide entertainment, although it is important to monitor their reactions to ensure they do not become stressed. Water play can be another enjoyable activity for bearded dragons. Many bearded dragons enjoy soaking in shallow water, and providing a small, safe water dish where they can splash around can be both fun and beneficial for their hydration and skin health. Some owners even report that their dragons enjoy gentle misting or being bathed in a shallow tub. This can also be an opportunity to bond with your dragon, as they may enjoy the interaction and attention.

Outdoor time, under controlled conditions, can be incredibly enriching for bearded dragons. Natural sunlight provides essential UVB rays that are crucial for their health, and the opportunity to explore a new environment can be very stimulating. Setting up a secure outdoor enclosure or using a reptile harness can allow your dragon to safely enjoy the outdoors. This can provide a variety of new sights, smells, and textures, which can be very exciting for them. However, it is important to supervise them closely to ensure their safety and prevent escape. Social interaction with their human caretakers is also a vital aspect of a bearded dragon's enrichment. Regular handling and gentle interaction can help build trust and strengthen the bond between you and your dragon. Activities such as hand-feeding, gentle petting, and allowing them to explore your surroundings under supervision can be very rewarding for both you and your dragon. It is important to approach these interactions with patience and care, respecting your dragon's comfort levels and ensuring they feel safe and secure.

Incorporating a variety of these activities into your bearded dragon's routine can help prevent boredom and promote a healthy, active lifestyle. Observing your dragon's reactions to different stimuli can also provide valuable insights into their preferences and personality, allowing you to tailor their enrichment activities to their individual needs. For example, some dragons may prefer more active pursuits like chasing a laser pointer, while others may enjoy the calm of soaking in a water dish or exploring a new environment. Understanding these preferences can help you create a more engaging and fulfilling environment for your dragon. Research and case studies have shown that environmental enrichment is crucial for the well-being of captive reptiles. Studies on other reptile species, such as iguanas and snakes, have demonstrated that providing a stimulating environment can reduce stress, improve physical health, and encourage natural behaviors. While specific research on bearded dragons is limited, these findings can be extrapolated to suggest that similar benefits can be achieved through appropriate enrichment activities.

In conclusion, providing a variety of engaging and stimulating activities is essential for the mental and physical well-being of bearded dragons. From interactive play and hunting live prey to environmental enrichment and social interaction, there are many ways to keep your dragon entertained and healthy. By understanding their natural behaviors and preferences, you can create a dynamic and enriching environment that promotes their overall happiness and well-being. Whether through the use of toys, outdoor exploration, or regular handling, the key is to offer a diverse range of activities that cater to their instincts and interests. This not only enhances their quality of life but also strengthens the bond between you and your scaly companion, making the journey of bearded dragon ownership a truly rewarding experience.

6. Handling and bonding

Handling and bonding with your bearded dragon is a crucial aspect of ensuring a happy and healthy relationship with your new scaly friend. This chapter will delve into the intricacies of safely handling your bearded dragon, building trust, and fostering a strong bond that will last throughout your pet's life. Understanding the importance of proper handling techniques is the first step in creating a positive experience for both you and your bearded dragon. When you first bring your bearded dragon home, it is essential to give them time to acclimate to their new environment. This period of adjustment is crucial for reducing stress and allowing your bearded dragon to feel secure. Start by observing your bearded dragon's behavior from a distance, allowing them to explore their habitat and become comfortable with their surroundings. During this initial phase, avoid handling your bearded dragon excessively, as this can cause unnecessary stress and hinder the bonding process.

Once your bearded dragon appears more relaxed and comfortable, you can begin the process of handling. Approach your bearded dragon slowly and calmly, speaking in a soft and reassuring tone. It is important to move gently and avoid sudden movements that may startle your pet. When picking up your bearded dragon, always support their body with both hands, ensuring that their entire weight is evenly distributed. One hand should be placed under their chest, just behind their front legs, while the other hand supports their hindquarters. This method of handling provides stability and prevents your bearded dragon from feeling insecure or threatened.

Consistency is key when it comes to handling your bearded dragon. Regular, gentle handling sessions will help your pet become accustomed to human interaction and build trust over time. Start with short handling sessions, gradually increasing the duration as your bearded dragon becomes more comfortable. It is important to pay attention to your bearded dragon's body language during these sessions. Signs of stress, such as puffing up, hissing, or attempting to escape, indicate that your bearded dragon may need a break. Respect their boundaries and allow them to return to their habitat if they show signs of discomfort.

Building trust with your bearded dragon is a gradual process that requires patience and consistency. One effective way to foster trust is through positive reinforcement. Offering treats during handling sessions can create a positive association with human interaction. Choose healthy, bearded dragon-friendly treats, such as small pieces of fruit or insects, and offer them as a reward for calm and cooperative behavior. Over time, your bearded dragon will learn to associate handling with positive experiences, making them more receptive to human interaction.

In addition to handling, spending quality time with your bearded dragon outside of their enclosure can strengthen your bond. Create a safe and controlled environment where your bearded dragon can explore and interact with you. This can be as simple as allowing them to roam a designated area of your home or setting up a playpen with various enrichment items. Supervised exploration provides mental stimulation and allows your bearded dragon to exercise their natural curiosity. During these sessions, continue to interact with your bearded dragon, offering gentle strokes and speaking in a soothing tone. This positive interaction reinforces the bond between you and your pet.

Understanding your bearded dragon's behavior is essential for successful bonding. Bearded dragons communicate through a variety of body language cues, and being able to interpret these signals will help you respond appropriately to their needs. For example, a bearded dragon that is feeling threatened or stressed may puff up their beard, darken their coloration, or flatten their body. On the other hand, a relaxed and content bearded dragon may exhibit behaviors such as basking, head bobbing, or arm waving. By paying attention to these cues, you can adjust your handling techniques and interactions to ensure your bearded dragon feels safe and secure.

Interactive activities can also play a significant role in bonding with your bearded dragon. Providing opportunities for mental and physical stimulation can enhance your pet's overall well-being and strengthen your relationship. Consider incorporating activities such as gentle play, puzzle feeders, or training sessions into your routine. Training your bearded dragon to perform simple tasks, such as coming when called or climbing onto your hand, can be a rewarding experience for both you and your pet. Use positive reinforcement techniques, such as treats and praise, to encourage desired behaviors and create a positive learning environment.

Handling do's and don'ts are important guidelines to follow to ensure the safety and well-being of your bearded dragon. Do handle your bearded dragon regularly to build trust and familiarity. Do support their body properly to prevent injury. Do observe their body language and respect their boundaries. Do provide positive reinforcement to create a positive association with handling. On the other hand, don't handle your bearded dragon if they are showing signs of stress or discomfort. Don't grab or squeeze your bearded dragon, as this can cause injury or fear. Don't handle your bearded dragon immediately after they have eaten, as this can lead to regurgitation. Don't leave your bearded dragon unattended during handling sessions, as this can result in accidents or escape.

Troubleshooting common issues that may arise during handling and bonding is an important aspect of being a responsible bearded dragon owner. If your bearded dragon is consistently displaying signs of stress or aggression during handling, it may be necessary to reassess your approach. Consider factors such as the handling environment, your handling techniques, and your bearded dragon's overall health and well-being. Consulting with a reptile veterinarian or an experienced reptile handler can provide valuable insights and guidance. Additionally, joining online forums or local reptile clubs can connect you with other bearded dragon enthusiasts who can offer support and advice.

In conclusion, handling and bonding with your bearded dragon is a rewarding and essential aspect of pet ownership. By following proper handling techniques, building trust through positive reinforcement, and understanding your bearded dragon's behavior, you can create a strong and lasting bond with your scaly companion. Remember to be patient, consistent, and attentive to your bearded dragon's needs. With time and effort, you will develop a deep and meaningful relationship that will bring joy and fulfillment to both you and your bearded dragon.

6.1 Introduction to handling

Handling a bearded dragon is an essential aspect of building a strong bond with your pet, and it begins with understanding the proper techniques to ensure both safety and comfort for your scaly friend. The first step in handling a bearded dragon is to approach them calmly and confidently. Sudden movements or loud noises can startle them, leading to stress or defensive behavior. When approaching your bearded dragon, it's crucial to move slowly and speak softly, allowing them to become accustomed to your presence. This initial approach sets the tone for a positive interaction and helps to build trust over time.

Once you are close to your bearded dragon, extend your hand slowly and allow them to see and smell you. Bearded dragons rely heavily on their sense of sight and smell to recognize their surroundings and the creatures within it. By allowing them to familiarize themselves with your scent, you are helping to reduce any anxiety they may feel. It's important to remember that each bearded dragon has its own personality and comfort level with handling, so patience is key. Some may be more curious and willing to interact, while others may take longer to warm up to you.

When you are ready to pick up your bearded dragon, it's essential to support their entire body. Place one hand under their chest, just behind their front legs, and use your other hand to support their hindquarters. This two-handed approach ensures that your bearded dragon feels secure and prevents any accidental falls or injuries. Avoid grabbing or squeezing your bearded dragon, as this can cause stress and discomfort. Instead, use a gentle but firm grip to lift them up and hold them close to your body. This proximity helps them feel more secure and less likely to squirm or try to escape.

It's also important to be mindful of your bearded dragon's body language during handling. Signs of stress or discomfort can include puffing up their beard, hissing, or trying to wriggle free. If you notice any of these behaviors, it's best to gently place your bearded dragon back in their enclosure and give them some time to calm down. Over time, as your bearded dragon becomes more accustomed to handling, these stress behaviors should decrease, and they will become more relaxed and comfortable in your hands.

Another key aspect of handling bearded dragons is to establish a routine. Regular handling sessions help your bearded dragon become more familiar with you and the process of being picked up and held. Start with short, daily handling sessions of just a few minutes, gradually increasing the duration as your bearded dragon becomes more comfortable. Consistency is crucial, as it helps to reinforce positive associations with handling and builds trust between you and your pet.

In addition to regular handling, it's important to create positive experiences for your bearded dragon during these sessions. This can include offering treats, gentle petting, or allowing them to explore a safe, enclosed area outside of their tank. Positive reinforcement helps to create a bond between you and your bearded dragon and makes handling a more enjoyable experience for both of you.

It's also worth noting that the time of day can impact your bearded dragon's receptiveness to handling. Bearded dragons are diurnal, meaning they are most active during the day and sleep at night. Handling them during their active periods, typically in the morning or early afternoon, can result in a more positive experience. Avoid handling your bearded dragon during their sleep or rest periods, as this can cause unnecessary stress and disrupt their natural rhythms.

For new bearded dragon owners, it can be helpful to observe experienced handlers or seek advice from reputable sources, such as books, online forums, or reptile care communities. Learning from others who have successfully handled bearded dragons can provide valuable insights and tips to improve your own handling techniques. Additionally, attending local reptile expos or pet clubs can offer opportunities to see handling demonstrations and ask questions from knowledgeable reptile enthusiasts.

In conclusion, handling a bearded dragon is a fundamental part of building a strong, trusting relationship with your pet. By approaching them calmly, supporting their entire body, and being mindful of their body language, you can create a positive handling experience that fosters trust and comfort. Establishing a routine, using positive reinforcement, and seeking advice from experienced handlers can further enhance your handling skills and ensure that your bearded dragon feels safe and secure in your care. With patience, consistency, and a gentle touch, you can develop a rewarding bond with your bearded dragon that will last a lifetime.

6.2 Understanding bearded dragon behavior

Understanding the behavior of bearded dragons is crucial for any owner aiming to build a strong bond and ensure the well-being of their scaly companion. These fascinating reptiles exhibit a range of behaviors that can provide insights into their comfort, stress levels, and overall health. By learning to read and interpret these behaviors, owners can create a more harmonious and enriching environment for their bearded dragons.

Bearded dragons, or Pogona vitticeps, are native to the arid regions of Australia. In the wild, they have developed a variety of behaviors to survive and thrive in their harsh environment. These behaviors are carried over into captivity and can be observed in pet bearded dragons. One of the most distinctive behaviors is the "beard puffing" or "beard display." When a bearded dragon feels threatened or is trying to assert dominance, it will puff out the skin around its throat, which turns black, giving the appearance of a larger, more intimidating creature. This behavior is often accompanied by an open mouth and a hissing sound. Understanding this display is essential for owners, as it indicates that the dragon is feeling threatened or stressed.

Another common behavior is arm-waving. This slow, circular motion of one of the front limbs is often seen in younger dragons or submissive individuals. It is a sign of submission and is used to communicate that the dragon is not a threat. This behavior can also be observed in interactions with other bearded dragons or even with humans. Recognizing arm-waving can help owners understand their pet's social dynamics and prevent unnecessary stress.

Head bobbing is another behavior that bearded dragons use to communicate. Rapid head bobbing is typically a sign of dominance or territoriality, often seen in males during the breeding season. Slower head bobs can be a sign of acknowledgment or a greeting. By paying attention to the context in which head bobbing occurs, owners can better understand their dragon's social interactions and mood.

Bearded dragons also exhibit a range of behaviors related to their thermoregulation needs. As ectothermic animals, they rely on external heat sources to regulate their body temperature. Basking is a behavior where the dragon positions itself under a heat source to absorb warmth. This is often accompanied by a flattened body posture to maximize surface area exposure. Conversely, when a bearded dragon is too warm, it may seek out cooler areas of the enclosure or exhibit behaviors such as gaping, where it opens its mouth to release excess heat. Understanding these thermoregulatory behaviors is crucial for maintaining an appropriate habitat and ensuring the dragon's comfort.

Feeding behaviors can also provide valuable insights into a bearded dragon's health and well-being. A healthy dragon will exhibit a strong feeding response, eagerly chasing down live prey or consuming vegetables and fruits. Changes in feeding behavior, such as a sudden lack of interest in food or difficulty eating, can be early indicators of health issues. Monitoring feeding behaviors and maintaining a consistent feeding schedule can help owners detect and address potential problems early.

Stress is a significant factor that can impact a bearded dragon's behavior. Signs of stress can include a lack of appetite, lethargy, frequent hiding, and changes in coloration. Stress can be caused by a variety of factors, including improper habitat conditions, handling, or the presence of other pets. By identifying and mitigating sources of stress, owners can help their bearded dragons lead healthier, happier lives.

One case study that highlights the importance of understanding bearded dragon behavior involves a dragon named Spike. Spike's owner noticed that he had become increasingly lethargic and was spending most of his time hiding. Initially, the owner attributed this behavior to normal brumation, a hibernation-like state that bearded dragons can enter during cooler months. However, upon closer observation, the owner noticed that Spike's coloration had become dull and he had lost interest in food. Concerned, the owner took Spike to a reptile veterinarian, who diagnosed him with a respiratory infection. The vet explained that the stress of improper humidity levels in Spike's enclosure had likely contributed to the infection. By understanding and recognizing the signs of stress and illness, Spike's owner was able to seek timely veterinary care and make necessary adjustments to the habitat, ultimately improving Spike's health and well-being.

In addition to recognizing signs of stress and illness, understanding bearded dragon behavior can enhance the bonding experience between the pet and its owner. Regular, gentle handling can help build trust and reduce stress. It's important to approach handling sessions with patience and to be attuned to the dragon's comfort levels. Signs that a bearded dragon is comfortable with handling include relaxed body posture, closed eyes, and a lack of defensive behaviors such as beard puffing or hissing. Over time, consistent and positive interactions can lead to a strong bond between the owner and the bearded dragon.

Interactive activities can also play a significant role in understanding and enriching a bearded dragon's behavior. Providing opportunities for exploration and mental stimulation can prevent boredom and promote natural behaviors. For example, placing a variety of objects in the enclosure, such as rocks, branches, and hides, can encourage climbing and basking behaviors. Additionally, allowing supervised out-of-enclosure time in a safe, controlled environment can provide further enrichment and exercise. Owners can also engage their bearded dragons with interactive feeding methods, such as using feeding tongs to simulate hunting or creating foraging opportunities with hidden food items.

Research has shown that environmental enrichment can have a positive impact on the behavior and well-being of captive reptiles. A study published in the journal "Applied Animal Behaviour Science" found that providing environmental enrichment, such as varied substrates and climbing structures, led to increased activity levels and reduced signs of stress in captive bearded dragons. This research underscores the importance of creating a stimulating and dynamic environment for pet bearded dragons.

Understanding bearded dragon behavior is a continuous learning process that requires observation, patience, and a willingness to adapt. Each bearded dragon is an individual with its own unique personality and preferences. By taking the time to learn and respond to these behaviors, owners can create a more fulfilling and harmonious relationship with their pets. Whether it's recognizing the subtle signs of stress, interpreting social behaviors, or providing enriching activities, understanding bearded dragon behavior is key to ensuring a happy, healthy, and well-adjusted pet.

In conclusion, understanding bearded dragon behavior is an essential aspect of responsible pet ownership. By learning to read and interpret the various behaviors exhibited by these fascinating reptiles, owners can create a more enriching and supportive environment for their pets. From recognizing signs of stress and illness to enhancing the bonding experience through positive interactions and enrichment, understanding bearded dragon behavior is a rewarding and ongoing journey. With patience, observation, and a commitment to continuous learning, owners can ensure that their bearded dragons lead happy, healthy, and fulfilling lives.

6.3 Bonding through routine

Establishing a consistent routine is a cornerstone in building trust and fostering a deeper bond with your bearded dragon. Much like humans, bearded dragons thrive on predictability and structure, which can significantly enhance their sense of security and well-being. The process of bonding through routine begins with understanding the natural rhythms and behaviors of your bearded dragon. In the wild, these reptiles have a set pattern of activities dictated by the cycle of day and night, temperature fluctuations, and availability of food. By mimicking these natural conditions in captivity, you can create an environment where your bearded dragon feels at ease and more inclined to interact positively with you.

Start by establishing a daily schedule that aligns with your bearded dragon's natural habits. This includes regular feeding times, consistent lighting schedules, and routine handling sessions. Feeding your bearded dragon at the same times each day helps them anticipate and look forward to meal times, which can be a bonding opportunity. For instance, if you feed your dragon in the morning and evening, ensure that these times are adhered to as closely as possible. This predictability not only aids in their digestion but also reinforces a sense of trust, as your dragon learns to associate you with positive experiences.

Lighting plays a crucial role in your bearded dragon's routine. Bearded dragons are diurnal, meaning they are active during the day and rest at night. Providing a consistent light cycle that mimics natural daylight hours helps regulate their biological clock. Typically, a 12-hour light and 12-hour dark cycle works well. Using timers for your lighting setup can ensure that this schedule remains consistent, even if you are not home. This consistency in lighting helps your bearded dragon know when to be active and when to rest, reducing stress and promoting a healthy lifestyle.

Handling your bearded dragon regularly is another critical aspect of building a bond through routine. Start with short, gentle handling sessions and gradually increase the duration as your dragon becomes more comfortable. Consistency is key here; try to handle your dragon at the same times each day. This could be in the morning after their basking session or in the evening before their lights go out. The goal is to make handling a predictable part of their day, so they come to expect and enjoy these interactions. Always approach your dragon calmly and confidently, as sudden movements or nervous handling can cause stress and hinder the bonding process.

Incorporating interactive activities into your routine can also strengthen the bond between you and your bearded dragon. These activities can include supervised exploration outside their enclosure, offering enrichment items like climbing branches or digging substrates, and even simple games like chasing a laser pointer. Each of these activities provides mental and physical stimulation, which is essential for your dragon's overall well-being. By engaging in these activities regularly, you not only keep your dragon active and healthy but also create positive associations with your presence.

Case studies have shown that bearded dragons respond well to routines that include regular interaction and enrichment. For example, a study conducted by reptile behaviorists found that bearded dragons who were handled and interacted with on a consistent schedule exhibited lower stress levels and were more likely to approach their owners voluntarily. This research underscores the importance of routine in fostering a trusting relationship with your bearded dragon.

It's also important to note that every bearded dragon is unique, and their preferences and comfort levels may vary. Pay close attention to your dragon's body language and behavior to gauge their response to the routine you establish. Signs of stress, such as darkened coloration, glass surfing, or refusal to eat, may indicate that adjustments are needed. Conversely, a relaxed posture, bright coloration, and active engagement in their environment are positive signs that your routine is effective.

In addition to daily routines, consider incorporating weekly and monthly activities that contribute to your bearded dragon's health and happiness. Weekly activities might include a warm bath to aid in hydration and shedding, while monthly activities could involve a thorough cleaning of their enclosure and a health check to monitor for any signs of illness. These activities, when performed regularly, not only ensure your dragon's well-being but also provide additional opportunities for bonding.

Building a bond through routine is a gradual process that requires patience and consistency. The more effort you put into establishing and maintaining a routine, the stronger your relationship with your bearded dragon will become. Over time, you will notice that your dragon becomes more responsive to your presence, more relaxed during handling, and more engaged in interactive activities. This bond is not only rewarding for you as a pet owner but also contributes to the overall health and happiness of your bearded dragon.

In conclusion, bonding with your bearded dragon through routine involves creating a predictable and structured environment that mimics their natural habits. By establishing regular feeding times, consistent lighting schedules, and routine handling sessions, you can build trust and foster a deeper connection with your dragon. Incorporating interactive activities and paying attention to your dragon's unique preferences further strengthens this bond. Remember, patience and consistency are key, and the effort you invest in creating a routine will be rewarded with a happy, healthy, and trusting bearded dragon.

6.4 Interactive activities

Interactive activities are essential for fostering a strong bond between you and your bearded dragon, enhancing their quality of life, and ensuring they remain mentally and physically stimulated. Engaging with your bearded dragon through various activities not only builds trust but also helps you understand their unique personality and preferences. One of the most straightforward yet effective interactive activities is gentle petting. Bearded dragons, like many reptiles, can be sensitive to touch, so it's crucial to approach them calmly and gently. Start by slowly extending your hand towards your dragon, allowing them to become familiar with your scent. Gradually, you can begin to stroke their back or under their chin, areas where they are generally more receptive to touch. Over time, this gentle petting can become a comforting routine that your bearded dragon looks forward to, reinforcing the bond between you.

Feeding by hand is another powerful way to connect with your bearded dragon. This activity not only provides nourishment but also serves as a trust-building exercise. Begin by offering small, manageable pieces of their favorite food, such as insects or vegetables, directly from your hand. This encourages your bearded dragon to associate your presence with positive experiences. As they become more comfortable, you can introduce more complex feeding interactions, such as using feeding tongs or placing food in different areas of their habitat to encourage exploration. Hand-feeding sessions can be particularly beneficial for new or shy dragons, helping them acclimate to their new environment and owner.

Supervised exploration outside the habitat is an excellent way to provide mental stimulation and physical exercise for your bearded dragon. Creating a safe, controlled environment for your dragon to explore can significantly enhance their well-being. Start by selecting a secure area free from potential hazards, such as other pets, small objects they could ingest, or areas where they could become trapped. Allow your bearded dragon to roam and investigate their surroundings at their own pace, always keeping a close eye on them to ensure their safety. This exploration time can be enriched with various stimuli, such as different textures to walk on, objects to climb, and even shallow water dishes for them to splash in. These activities mimic their natural behaviors and environments, promoting physical health and mental engagement.

Interactive play sessions can also include the use of toys and enrichment items. While bearded dragons may not play with toys in the same way as mammals, they can still benefit from items that stimulate their natural instincts. For example, small balls or crumpled paper can be intriguing objects for them to push around with their nose or claws. Mirrors can also be fascinating for bearded dragons, as they may react to their reflection, thinking it is another dragon. However, it's essential to monitor their reactions closely, as some dragons may become stressed or aggressive when confronted with their reflection. Rotating these enrichment items regularly keeps the environment fresh and exciting, preventing boredom and promoting a more active lifestyle.

Another engaging activity is training your bearded dragon to perform simple tasks or tricks. While this may sound ambitious, bearded dragons are capable of learning through positive reinforcement. Start with basic commands, such as coming to you when called or following a target, like a brightly colored stick. Use treats as rewards to reinforce positive behavior. Training sessions should be short and consistent, focusing on one task at a time to avoid overwhelming your dragon. Over time, these training exercises can become a fun and rewarding way to interact with your pet, strengthening your bond and providing mental stimulation.

Case studies have shown that bearded dragons who engage in regular interactive activities tend to be more active, exhibit fewer signs of stress, and have better overall health. For instance, a study conducted by reptile behaviorists found that bearded dragons provided with daily enrichment activities, such as supervised exploration and interactive feeding, displayed more natural behaviors and had lower stress levels compared to those kept in more static environments. This research underscores the importance of incorporating a variety of interactive activities into your bearded dragon's routine.

In addition to these activities, it's crucial to pay attention to your bearded dragon's body language and signals. Each dragon is unique, and what works for one may not be suitable for another. Observing their reactions to different activities can help you tailor your interactions to their preferences, ensuring a positive and enriching experience. For example, if your dragon seems stressed or disinterested in a particular activity, it's essential to respect their boundaries and try a different approach.

Interactive activities are not just about keeping your bearded dragon entertained; they are about building a deep, trusting relationship. By investing time and effort into these activities, you create a bond that goes beyond mere pet ownership. Your bearded dragon will come to recognize you as a source of comfort, security, and enrichment, leading to a happier and healthier life for both of you. Whether through gentle petting, hand-feeding, supervised exploration, or training, these interactions are the foundation of a fulfilling and rewarding relationship with your bearded dragon.

6.5 Handling do's and don'ts

When it comes to handling your bearded dragon, understanding the essential do's and don'ts is crucial for ensuring both your safety and the well-being of your pet. Handling a bearded dragon is not just about picking them up and carrying them around; it involves a series of careful steps and considerations that help build trust and foster a strong bond between you and your scaly companion. Let's delve into the intricacies of handling your bearded dragon, supported by examples, case studies, and research to provide a comprehensive guide.

First and foremost, always approach your bearded dragon calmly and gently. Sudden movements or loud noises can startle them, leading to stress or defensive behavior. When you reach out to pick up your bearded dragon, do so from the side rather than from above. In the wild, predators often attack from above, so approaching from the side is less threatening and helps your bearded dragon feel more secure. Use both hands to support their body, ensuring that their entire weight is evenly distributed. One hand should be placed under their chest, just behind the front legs, while the other hand supports their hindquarters. This method provides stability and prevents any accidental falls or injuries.

It's important to handle your bearded dragon regularly but not excessively. Regular handling helps them become accustomed to human interaction and reduces stress over time. However, over-handling can lead to stress and fatigue, especially in younger or newly acquired bearded dragons. Start with short handling sessions, gradually increasing the duration as your bearded dragon becomes more comfortable. Aim for handling sessions of about 10-15 minutes initially, and observe your pet's behavior closely. Signs of stress, such as rapid breathing, darkening of the beard, or attempts to escape, indicate that it's time to return your bearded dragon to its enclosure.

One of the key do's of handling is to always wash your hands before and after each session. Bearded dragons can carry Salmonella bacteria, which can be transmitted to humans. Washing your hands with soap and water helps prevent the spread of bacteria and ensures good hygiene. Additionally, avoid handling your bearded dragon if you have any open cuts or wounds on your hands, as this increases the risk of infection.

When handling your bearded dragon, it's essential to provide a secure and comfortable environment. Avoid handling them in high-traffic areas or places with loud noises, as these can cause unnecessary stress. Instead, choose a quiet and calm location where your bearded dragon can feel safe. If you're handling your bearded dragon outside of their enclosure, ensure that the area is free of potential hazards, such as other pets, sharp objects, or small spaces where your bearded dragon could get stuck.

Another important aspect of handling is to be mindful of your bearded dragon's body language. Bearded dragons communicate their comfort levels through various physical cues. For example, a relaxed bearded dragon will have a calm demeanor, with its limbs resting comfortably and its eyes open. On the other hand, a stressed or frightened bearded dragon may puff up its beard, flatten its body, or try to escape. By paying attention to these cues, you can adjust your handling approach to ensure your bearded dragon remains comfortable and stress-free.

It's also crucial to avoid certain don'ts when handling your bearded dragon. Never grab your bearded dragon by the tail, as this can cause severe injury or even lead to tail autotomy, where the tail breaks off as a defense mechanism. Additionally, avoid squeezing or applying excessive pressure to your bearded dragon's body, as this can cause internal injuries. Be gentle and supportive, allowing your bearded dragon to move freely while in your hands.

One common mistake new bearded dragon owners make is handling their pet immediately after feeding. Bearded dragons need time to digest their food, and handling them too soon after a meal can lead to regurgitation or digestive issues. Wait at least an hour after feeding before handling your bearded dragon to ensure their digestive system is not disrupted.

Case studies have shown that proper handling techniques can significantly impact a bearded dragon's overall well-being and behavior. For example, a study conducted by reptile behaviorists found that bearded dragons handled gently and regularly exhibited lower stress levels and were more likely to engage in positive social interactions with their owners. In contrast, bearded dragons that were handled roughly or infrequently showed higher levels of stress and were more prone to defensive behaviors.

Interactive activities can also enhance the handling experience for both you and your bearded dragon. Incorporate gentle petting and stroking into your handling sessions, focusing on areas where your bearded dragon enjoys being touched, such as the top of their head or along their back. You can also use handling sessions as an opportunity for enrichment by allowing your bearded dragon to explore different textures and surfaces, such as soft towels or grassy areas. This not only provides mental stimulation but also helps your bearded dragon become more comfortable with various environments.

Troubleshooting common issues related to handling is an essential part of the process. If your bearded dragon consistently shows signs of stress during handling, consider evaluating your approach. Are you handling them too frequently or for too long? Are there environmental factors, such as loud noises or other pets, that could be causing stress? Adjusting these factors can help create a more positive handling experience. Additionally, if your bearded dragon exhibits aggressive behavior, such as biting or hissing, it's important to address the underlying cause. This could be due to fear, discomfort, or territorial instincts. Gradual desensitization and positive reinforcement can help reduce aggressive behavior over time.

In conclusion, handling your bearded dragon with care and consideration is essential for building a strong bond and ensuring their well-being. By following the do's and avoiding the don'ts of handling, you can create a positive and enriching experience for both you and your bearded dragon. Remember to approach your bearded dragon calmly, support their body properly, and be mindful of their body language. Regular, gentle handling sessions, combined with good hygiene practices and a secure environment, will help your bearded dragon feel safe and comfortable. With patience and consistency, you can foster a trusting and rewarding relationship with your bearded dragon, enhancing the joy and fulfillment of owning this unique and fascinating pet.

6.6 Troubleshooting common issues

Troubleshooting common issues in handling and bonding with your bearded dragon can be a challenging yet rewarding aspect of pet ownership. As a new owner, you may encounter various hurdles that can affect the relationship between you and your scaly companion. Understanding these potential issues and knowing how to address them is crucial for fostering a healthy and trusting bond. One of the most common issues is the initial fear and stress that a bearded dragon might experience when first introduced to a new environment. This can manifest in behaviors such as hiding, refusing to eat, or displaying defensive postures like puffing up their beard and hissing. To mitigate this, it is essential to give your bearded dragon time to acclimate to their new surroundings. Gradually introduce handling sessions, starting with short, gentle interactions and slowly increasing the duration as your pet becomes more comfortable. Patience is key, as forcing interactions can exacerbate stress and hinder the bonding process.

Another frequent challenge is the bearded dragon's reluctance to be handled. This can be due to various factors, including previous negative experiences, improper handling techniques, or simply the dragon's individual temperament. To address this, ensure that you are approaching your bearded dragon calmly and confidently. Sudden movements or loud noises can startle them, making them more resistant to handling. Always support their body fully, using both hands to gently lift them from underneath. Consistency in handling routines can also help build trust. For example, handling your bearded dragon at the same time each day can create a sense of predictability and security. Additionally, offering treats during or after handling sessions can create positive associations with being held.

Health issues can also impact the handling and bonding process. Bearded dragons suffering from ailments such as metabolic bone disease, respiratory infections, or parasites may be more irritable and less willing to be handled. Regular veterinary check-ups are crucial to ensure your pet's health and well-being. If you notice any signs of illness, such as lethargy, weight loss, or abnormal stool, seek veterinary care promptly. Addressing health issues not only improves your bearded dragon's quality of life but also makes them more receptive to handling and bonding.

Environmental factors play a significant role in your bearded dragon's behavior and willingness to bond. Inadequate habitat conditions, such as incorrect temperature gradients, insufficient UVB lighting, or improper substrate, can cause stress and discomfort. Ensure that your bearded dragon's enclosure mimics their natural habitat as closely as possible. This includes providing appropriate basking and cool areas, maintaining proper humidity levels, and offering hiding spots for security. A well-maintained habitat promotes a sense of well-being, making your bearded dragon more likely to engage positively with you.

Behavioral issues can also arise from misunderstandings of your bearded dragon's body language and social cues. For instance, a bearded dragon that is waving its arm may be signaling submission or stress, while head bobbing can indicate dominance or territorial behavior. Learning to interpret these signals accurately can help you respond appropriately and avoid actions that might cause distress. Observing your bearded dragon's behavior during interactions can provide valuable insights into their comfort levels and preferences.

Case studies have shown that individual bearded dragons can have unique personalities and bonding experiences. For example, one owner reported that their bearded dragon, initially very skittish and defensive, gradually became more trusting through consistent, gentle handling and positive reinforcement with treats. Over time, the dragon began to seek out interaction and even enjoyed being petted. Another owner found success by incorporating interactive activities, such as letting their bearded dragon explore a safe, enclosed space outside the enclosure, which provided mental stimulation and strengthened their bond.

Research supports the importance of routine and consistency in building trust with reptiles. A study published in the Journal of Herpetology found that reptiles, including bearded dragons, exhibit reduced stress levels when handled regularly and predictably. This underscores the significance of establishing a routine that your bearded dragon can rely on, which in turn fosters a sense of security and trust.

In conclusion, troubleshooting common issues in handling and bonding with your bearded dragon requires a combination of patience, understanding, and consistent care. By addressing environmental, health, and behavioral factors, and by learning to interpret your bearded dragon's signals, you can overcome challenges and build a strong, trusting relationship with your pet. Remember that each bearded dragon is an individual, and what works for one may not work for another. Stay observant, flexible, and committed to providing the best care possible, and you will be rewarded with a happy, healthy, and well-bonded bearded dragon.

7. Breeding and lifecycle

Breeding and lifecycle of bearded dragons is a fascinating and intricate process that requires a deep understanding of their natural behaviors, environmental needs, and developmental stages. The journey begins with understanding the breeding process, which is a critical aspect for anyone looking to breed these reptiles successfully. Bearded dragons reach sexual maturity at around 18 months to 2 years of age. The breeding season typically aligns with the warmer months, mimicking their natural habitat conditions in the wild. During this time, males exhibit pronounced behaviors such as head bobbing, beard darkening, and arm waving to attract females. It's essential to ensure that both the male and female are healthy and of appropriate size before attempting to breed them. The breeding process involves introducing the male to the female's enclosure, where he will perform a series of courtship behaviors. If the female is receptive, she will allow the male to mount her, and copulation will occur. After successful mating, the female will begin to show signs of gravidity, such as increased appetite and a noticeable bulge in her abdomen.

Egg laying and incubation are the next critical stages in the breeding process. A gravid female will require a suitable laying site, which can be provided by a lay box filled with a moist substrate such as vermiculite or sand. The female will dig a burrow to deposit her eggs, which can range from 15 to 30 in a single clutch. Once the eggs are laid, they need to be carefully removed and placed in an incubation container with a consistent temperature of around 82-86°F and a humidity level of 75-80%. The incubation period lasts approximately 60-80 days, during which the eggs must be monitored regularly to ensure they remain viable.

Hatchling care is a delicate and crucial phase that requires meticulous attention. Once the eggs hatch, the tiny bearded dragons emerge and should be placed in a separate enclosure with appropriate heating, lighting, and humidity levels. Hatchlings are highly vulnerable and require a diet rich in protein to support their rapid growth. Feeding them small insects such as pinhead crickets and finely chopped vegetables is essential. It's also important to provide a shallow water dish and ensure the enclosure is kept clean to prevent any health issues.

As the hatchlings grow, they enter the juvenile growth stages, which span from a few weeks old to around 6 months. During this period, they experience rapid growth and require a diet that supports their development. Juveniles should be fed multiple times a day with a variety of insects and vegetables to ensure they receive all the necessary nutrients. Regular handling and interaction are also important to help them become accustomed to human presence and reduce stress.

Adult bearded dragon health and maintenance involve providing a stable and enriching environment that mimics their natural habitat. Adults require a balanced diet that includes a mix of insects, vegetables, and occasional fruits. It's crucial to maintain proper temperature gradients within the enclosure, with a basking spot of around 95-110°F and a cooler area of 75-85°F. Regular health checks, including monitoring for signs of illness or stress, are essential to ensure the well-being of the adult bearded dragon.

Senior bearded dragon care focuses on addressing the specific needs of aging reptiles. As bearded dragons age, they may experience a decline in activity levels and changes in appetite. It's important to adjust their diet to include easily digestible foods and ensure they receive adequate hydration. Regular veterinary check-ups become increasingly important to monitor for age-related health issues such as metabolic bone disease or arthritis. Providing a comfortable and stress-free environment with appropriate lighting and temperature is crucial for the well-being of senior bearded dragons.

Understanding the breeding and lifecycle of bearded dragons is a rewarding experience that requires dedication and knowledge. Each stage, from breeding to caring for hatchlings, juveniles, adults, and seniors, presents unique challenges and responsibilities. By providing the appropriate care and environment at each stage, you can ensure the health and happiness of your bearded dragons throughout their lives. This comprehensive understanding of their lifecycle not only enhances your ability to care for them but also deepens your appreciation for these remarkable reptiles.

7.1 Understanding bearded dragon breeding

Understanding the breeding process of bearded dragons is a fascinating and intricate aspect of their care that requires a deep dive into their natural behaviors, ideal conditions for mating, and the preparatory steps necessary to ensure successful reproduction. Bearded dragons, scientifically known as Pogona, are native to the arid regions of Australia, where their breeding behaviors have evolved to adapt to the harsh environmental conditions. In captivity, replicating these conditions as closely as possible is crucial for encouraging natural breeding behaviors and ensuring the health and well-being of both the breeding pair and their offspring.

Mating behaviors in bearded dragons are a complex dance of visual and physical cues. Males typically initiate the courtship process through a series of head bobs, arm waves, and displays of their vibrant beards, which darken to a striking black color. These behaviors are not merely for show; they serve as signals to the female of the male's readiness and suitability as a mate. Females, in turn, respond with their own set of behaviors, such as slow head bobs and submissive postures, indicating their receptiveness to the male's advances. Understanding these behaviors is essential for breeders, as it allows them to recognize when their dragons are ready to mate and to intervene if necessary to prevent aggression or stress.

Ideal breeding conditions for bearded dragons involve carefully controlled environmental factors, including temperature, lighting, and habitat setup. In the wild, bearded dragons breed during the warmer months when food is abundant, and the conditions are optimal for raising young. To mimic this in captivity, breeders must ensure that the enclosure provides a temperature gradient, with basking spots reaching up to 110°F and cooler areas around 80°F. Additionally, providing a photoperiod that simulates natural daylight cycles, with 12-14 hours of light per day, helps to trigger the breeding cycle. The use of full-spectrum UVB lighting is also essential, as it promotes healthy calcium metabolism and overall well-being, which are critical for successful reproduction.

Preparing bearded dragons for breeding involves more than just creating the right environmental conditions; it also requires ensuring that both the male and female are in optimal health. This includes a well-balanced diet rich in calcium and vitamins, regular health checks to rule out any underlying conditions, and maintaining a stress-free environment. Female bearded dragons, in particular, need to be in peak physical condition, as the process of producing and laying eggs is physically demanding. Providing calcium supplements and ensuring proper hydration are vital steps in preparing the female for the rigors of egg production.

Once the breeding pair has successfully mated, the female will begin the process of developing eggs, known as gravidity. This period typically lasts between 4-6 weeks, during which the female's abdomen will noticeably swell as the eggs develop. During this time, it is crucial to provide the female with a diet high in calcium and protein to support the growing eggs. Additionally, offering a suitable laying site, such as a nesting box filled with a moist substrate like vermiculite or sand, is essential for the female to lay her eggs comfortably. The nesting box should be placed in a warm, quiet area of the enclosure to minimize stress and encourage the female to lay her eggs.

Once the eggs are laid, they must be carefully removed and placed in an incubator set to a temperature of around 82-86°F with a humidity level of 75-80%. The incubation period for bearded dragon eggs typically lasts between 55-75 days, during which the eggs must be monitored regularly to ensure they remain at the correct temperature and humidity levels. Any fluctuations in these conditions can negatively impact the development of the embryos, leading to deformities or failure to hatch.

Throughout the breeding process, it is essential to keep detailed records of mating dates, egg laying, and incubation conditions. This information is invaluable for tracking the success of breeding attempts and making any necessary adjustments to improve future outcomes. Additionally, maintaining accurate records helps to identify any potential health issues early on and ensures that the breeding pair and their offspring receive the best possible care.

In conclusion, understanding bearded dragon breeding requires a comprehensive approach that encompasses knowledge of their natural behaviors, ideal environmental conditions, and meticulous preparation and care. By replicating the conditions of their native habitat and providing the necessary support, breeders can successfully navigate the complexities of bearded dragon reproduction and contribute to the health and vitality of these captivating reptiles.

7.2 Egg laying and incubation

The egg-laying process in bearded dragons is a fascinating and intricate aspect of their reproductive cycle, requiring careful attention and precise conditions to ensure the healthy development of the eggs. Female bearded dragons, or gravid dragons, typically begin showing signs of pregnancy, such as increased appetite, noticeable weight gain, and a more pronounced belly. As the eggs develop within her, the female will exhibit nesting behaviors, such as digging and scratching at the substrate. This is a crucial time for the owner to prepare an appropriate laying area to accommodate her needs.

Creating a suitable egg-laying area involves providing a nesting box filled with a moist substrate, such as a mixture of sand and soil, which allows the female to dig and lay her eggs comfortably. The substrate should be kept at a consistent moisture level to prevent the eggs from drying out. The nesting box should be placed in a quiet, undisturbed area of the enclosure to reduce stress for the gravid female. Once the female is ready to lay her eggs, she will dig a burrow in the substrate, deposit the eggs, and then cover them up before leaving the nesting area.

After the eggs have been laid, it is essential to carefully remove them from the nesting box and transfer them to an incubation setup. This process should be done with great care to avoid damaging the delicate eggs. The eggs should be handled gently and placed in an incubation container filled with a suitable incubation medium, such as vermiculite or perlite, which helps maintain the necessary humidity levels. The eggs should be partially buried in the medium, with enough space between them to allow for proper air circulation.

The incubation container should then be placed in an incubator set to the appropriate temperature and humidity levels. Bearded dragon eggs typically require an incubation temperature of around 82-86°F (28-30°C) and a humidity level of 75-80%. Maintaining these conditions is critical for the healthy development of the embryos. It is important to monitor the temperature and humidity levels regularly and make any necessary adjustments to ensure a stable environment.

Throughout the incubation period, which usually lasts between 55 to 75 days, the eggs should be checked periodically for signs of mold or other issues. Any eggs that appear discolored, shriveled, or moldy should be removed to prevent contamination of the remaining eggs. As the incubation period progresses, the eggs will begin to show signs of development, such as increased size and slight changes in color.

Hatching is an exciting and delicate phase in the breeding process. As the embryos near the end of their development, they will start to absorb the remaining yolk sac, which provides essential nutrients for their growth. The hatchlings will then use a specialized egg tooth to break through the eggshell, a process known as pipping. It is crucial to allow the hatchlings to emerge from the eggs on their own, as intervening can cause harm to the delicate newborns.

Once the hatchlings have fully emerged, they should be transferred to a separate enclosure designed specifically for their needs. This enclosure should have appropriate heating, lighting, and substrate to support their growth and development. Hatchlings require a higher temperature gradient than adults, with a basking spot of around 105-110°F (40-43°C) and a cooler area of 80-85°F (27-29°C). Proper UVB lighting is also essential for their bone development and overall health.

Feeding hatchlings can be challenging, as they have small appetites and require a diet rich in protein and calcium to support their rapid growth. Offering a variety of appropriately sized insects, such as pinhead crickets and small dubia roaches, along with finely chopped vegetables, can help ensure they receive the necessary nutrients. It is also important to dust their food with calcium and vitamin supplements to prevent deficiencies.

In addition to providing the right diet, maintaining proper hydration is crucial for hatchlings. A shallow water dish should be available at all times, and the enclosure should be misted lightly to provide additional humidity. Monitoring the hatchlings' growth and health is essential, as any signs of illness or developmental issues should be addressed promptly with the help of a reptile veterinarian.

The egg-laying and incubation process in bearded dragons is a complex and rewarding experience that requires careful planning and attention to detail. By providing the right conditions and care, owners can ensure the successful development and hatching of healthy bearded dragon offspring. This journey not only deepens the bond between the owner and their bearded dragons but also contributes to the understanding and appreciation of these remarkable reptiles.

7.3 Hatchling care

Caring for hatchling bearded dragons is a meticulous yet rewarding endeavor that requires a deep understanding of their specific needs from the moment they emerge from their eggs. Hatchlings, being incredibly delicate, demand a precise environment to ensure their survival and healthy growth. One of the most critical aspects of hatchling care is maintaining the appropriate temperature within their enclosure. Hatchlings thrive in a controlled environment where the basking spot temperature is kept between 105-110°F (40-43°C), while the cooler side of the enclosure should be around 80-85°F (27-29°C). This gradient allows the hatchlings to thermoregulate, ensuring they can digest food properly and maintain optimal metabolic functions. A high-quality thermostat is essential to prevent temperature fluctuations that could stress or harm the young dragons.

Feeding protocols for hatchlings are equally crucial. Unlike adult bearded dragons, hatchlings require frequent feeding due to their rapid growth and high metabolic rate. They should be fed small insects, such as appropriately sized crickets or dubia roaches, multiple times a day. The insects should be no larger than the space between the hatchling's eyes to prevent choking or digestive issues. Additionally, offering finely chopped vegetables and greens is essential to introduce them to a varied diet early on. Calcium and vitamin D3 supplements should be dusted on their food several times a week to support bone development and prevent metabolic bone disease, a common ailment in young reptiles.

Initial health checks are vital to identify any potential issues early. Upon hatching, each dragon should be observed for signs of physical deformities, such as kinked tails or malformed limbs, which could indicate genetic issues or incubation problems. Regular monitoring for signs of illness, such as lethargy, lack of appetite, or abnormal feces, is necessary. A fecal exam by a reptile veterinarian can help detect parasites, which are common in hatchlings and can severely impact their health if left untreated. Ensuring proper hydration is another critical aspect of hatchling care. Hatchlings can become dehydrated quickly, so providing a shallow water dish and misting the enclosure lightly can help maintain adequate humidity levels. However, it is important to avoid excessive moisture, which can lead to respiratory issues.

Creating a stress-free environment is paramount for the well-being of hatchling bearded dragons. The enclosure should be set up with multiple hiding spots to allow the young dragons to feel secure.

Overhandling should be avoided during the first few weeks to minimize stress and allow the hatchlings to acclimate to their new surroundings. Gradual, gentle handling can be introduced as they grow and become more accustomed to human interaction. Lighting is another critical component of hatchling care. UVB lighting is essential for the synthesis of vitamin D3, which aids in calcium absorption. A high-quality UVB bulb should be installed and replaced every six months to ensure consistent exposure. The light cycle should mimic natural daylight, with 12-14 hours of light followed by 10-12 hours of darkness.

Case studies have shown that hatchlings raised in environments with optimal conditions and proper care protocols exhibit better growth rates, stronger immune systems, and overall improved health outcomes. For instance, a study conducted by reptile experts at a leading herpetology institute found that hatchlings provided with a balanced diet, appropriate supplementation, and a stable environment had a significantly lower incidence of metabolic bone disease and other common health issues compared to those raised in suboptimal conditions.

In conclusion, caring for hatchling bearded dragons requires a comprehensive approach that addresses their unique needs from temperature regulation and feeding to hydration and health monitoring. By providing a meticulously maintained environment and adhering to best practices in hatchling care, new owners can ensure their young bearded dragons thrive and develop into healthy adults. This journey, while demanding, is incredibly fulfilling and sets the foundation for a lifelong bond with these fascinating reptiles.

7.4 Juvenile growth stages

Understanding the growth phases of juvenile bearded dragons is crucial for ensuring their healthy development and well-being. Juvenile bearded dragons, typically ranging from one month to six months old, undergo significant changes in their physical and behavioral characteristics. During this period, they experience rapid growth, which necessitates adjustments in their diet, habitat, and overall care. As a new owner, it is essential to recognize and adapt to these changes to provide the best possible environment for your young bearded dragon.

In the initial stages of their juvenile phase, bearded dragons exhibit a high growth rate, often doubling in size within a few months. This rapid growth demands a diet rich in protein to support their developing muscles and bones. Insects such as crickets, mealworms, and dubia roaches should form the bulk of their diet, supplemented with a variety of leafy greens and vegetables to ensure a balanced intake of nutrients. It is important to dust these insects with calcium and vitamin D3 supplements to prevent metabolic bone disease, a common ailment in growing reptiles. As they grow, the frequency and quantity of feedings should be adjusted accordingly. Juvenile bearded dragons typically require multiple feedings per day, gradually transitioning to fewer feedings as they approach adulthood.

The habitat of a juvenile bearded dragon must also evolve to accommodate their increasing size and activity levels. A spacious tank with ample room for exploration and exercise is essential. As they grow, it may be necessary to upgrade to a larger enclosure to prevent overcrowding and stress. The tank should be equipped with appropriate lighting, including UVB and basking lights, to support their metabolic processes and overall health. The temperature gradient within the tank should be carefully monitored, with a basking area maintained at around 95-110°F and a cooler area at 75-85°F. This allows the juvenile dragon to thermoregulate effectively, promoting proper digestion and activity levels.

Behaviorally, juvenile bearded dragons are more active and curious compared to their adult counterparts. They require mental stimulation and opportunities for physical exercise to prevent boredom and promote healthy development. Providing a variety of climbing structures, hides, and interactive toys can help keep them engaged and reduce stress. Regular handling and interaction with your juvenile dragon can also aid in building trust and socialization, making them more comfortable with human contact as they mature.

Case studies have shown that juvenile bearded dragons raised in enriched environments with proper diet and care exhibit better growth rates and overall health compared to those in suboptimal conditions. For instance, a study conducted by reptile experts at the University of California found that juvenile bearded dragons provided with a varied diet and adequate UVB exposure had significantly higher bone density and muscle mass than those with limited dietary options and insufficient lighting. This highlights the importance of a holistic approach to their care, encompassing diet, habitat, and behavioral enrichment.

As your juvenile bearded dragon continues to grow, it is important to regularly assess their health and development. Regular veterinary check-ups can help identify any potential issues early on and ensure they receive appropriate care. Monitoring their weight, appetite, and activity levels can provide valuable insights into their overall well-being. Any sudden changes in behavior or physical appearance should be addressed promptly to prevent potential health problems.

In conclusion, understanding the growth phases of juvenile bearded dragons and adapting their care accordingly is essential for their healthy development. By providing a balanced diet, a spacious and well-equipped habitat, and opportunities for mental and physical stimulation, you can ensure your young bearded dragon thrives during this critical stage of their life. With proper care and attention, your juvenile bearded dragon will grow into a healthy and happy adult, ready to embark on the next phase of their journey with you.

7.5 Adult bearded dragon health and maintenance

As bearded dragons transition from their juvenile stages into adulthood, their care requirements evolve significantly, necessitating a nuanced understanding of their diet, habitat maintenance, and common health issues. Adult bearded dragons, typically defined as those over 18 months old, exhibit a range of behaviors and physiological needs that differ from their younger counterparts. One of the most critical aspects of adult bearded dragon care is their diet. Unlike juveniles, who require a diet rich in protein to support rapid growth, adults need a balanced diet that includes a higher proportion of vegetables and greens. A typical adult bearded dragon's diet should consist of approximately 70-80% vegetables and greens, with the remaining 20-30% comprising insects and other protein sources. Leafy greens such as collard greens, mustard greens, and dandelion greens are excellent choices, providing essential vitamins and minerals. Additionally, a variety of vegetables like bell peppers, squash, and carrots can be included to ensure a well-rounded diet. Protein sources should primarily include gut-loaded insects such as crickets, dubia roaches, and occasional treats like mealworms or superworms. It is crucial to dust these insects with calcium and vitamin D3 supplements to prevent metabolic bone disease, a common ailment in bearded dragons caused by calcium deficiency.

Habitat maintenance for adult bearded dragons also requires careful attention. As they grow, their need for space increases, and a tank size of at least 40 gallons is recommended, though larger tanks are preferable to allow for ample movement and enrichment. The substrate should be chosen with care to prevent impaction, a condition where indigestible materials block the digestive tract. Options such as reptile carpet, tile, or paper towels are safe and easy to clean. Temperature regulation remains vital, with a basking spot maintained at 95-105°F and a cooler area around 75-85°F. Proper lighting, including UVB light, is essential for calcium metabolism and overall health. The UVB light should be replaced every six months to ensure it provides adequate radiation. Additionally, providing hides and climbing structures can help mimic their natural environment, promoting physical and mental stimulation.

Common health issues in adult bearded dragons can range from metabolic bone disease and impaction to respiratory infections and parasites. Regular health checks are imperative to catch any signs of illness early. Symptoms such as lethargy, lack of appetite, abnormal stool, or respiratory distress should prompt immediate veterinary consultation. Preventive care strategies include maintaining a clean habitat, providing a balanced diet, and ensuring proper hydration. Bearded dragons can be prone to dehydration, so offering a shallow water dish and misting their enclosure can help maintain adequate moisture levels. Additionally, regular baths can aid in hydration and shedding.

Case studies have shown that bearded dragons with well-maintained habitats and balanced diets tend to have fewer health issues and longer lifespans. For instance, a study conducted by the Reptile Health and Welfare Institute found that bearded dragons kept in enclosures with proper temperature gradients, UVB lighting, and a varied diet had a 30% lower incidence of metabolic bone disease compared to those in suboptimal conditions. Another example involves a bearded dragon named Spike, who suffered from repeated impaction due to sand substrate. After switching to reptile carpet and adjusting his diet to include more leafy greens and properly sized insects, Spike's health improved significantly, and he no longer experienced digestive issues.

In conclusion, the care of adult bearded dragons requires a comprehensive approach that addresses their dietary needs, habitat maintenance, and potential health issues. By providing a balanced diet rich in vegetables and appropriately supplemented protein, maintaining a clean and adequately sized habitat with proper temperature and lighting, and staying vigilant for signs of illness, bearded dragon owners can ensure their pets lead healthy and fulfilling lives. As with any pet, the key to successful care lies in understanding their unique needs and being proactive in addressing them. Through diligent care and attention, adult bearded dragons can thrive, bringing joy and companionship to their owners for many years.

7.6 Senior bearded dragon care

As bearded dragons age, their care requirements evolve significantly, necessitating a tailored approach to ensure their well-being and comfort in their senior years. Understanding the unique needs of senior bearded dragons is crucial for any responsible pet owner, as it involves making dietary adjustments, closely monitoring their health, and managing their comfort to accommodate the natural changes that come with aging. Typically, bearded dragons are considered seniors when they reach around 7-8 years of age, though this can vary depending on individual health and genetics. One of the primary considerations for senior bearded dragons is their diet. As they age, their metabolism slows down, and their dietary needs shift. While younger dragons thrive on a diet rich in protein to support their rapid growth, senior dragons require a diet that is lower in protein and higher in fiber to support their digestive health. This means incorporating more leafy greens and vegetables while reducing the frequency of insect feedings. For example, collard greens, mustard greens, and dandelion greens are excellent choices, as they provide essential nutrients without the high protein content that could strain an older dragon's kidneys. Additionally, it's important to ensure that their food is easy to digest; finely chopping or even lightly steaming vegetables can make them more palatable and easier on an aging digestive system.

Health monitoring becomes increasingly vital as bearded dragons age. Regular veterinary check-ups are essential to catch any potential health issues early. Common health concerns in senior bearded dragons include metabolic bone disease, arthritis, and dental problems. Metabolic bone disease, often caused by a lack of calcium or improper UVB lighting, can be particularly problematic in older dragons. Ensuring they have access to adequate UVB lighting and providing calcium supplements can help mitigate this risk. Arthritis is another common issue, leading to stiffness and reduced mobility. Providing a comfortable habitat with easy-to-navigate terrain and soft substrates can help alleviate some of the discomfort associated with arthritis. Dental health is also a concern, as older dragons may experience tooth decay or gum disease. Regularly inspecting their mouths and providing appropriate chewable items can help maintain dental health.

Comfort management is another critical aspect of caring for senior bearded dragons. As they age, they may become less active and more prone to stress. Creating a serene and stress-free environment is essential. This includes maintaining optimal temperature gradients within their enclosure, as older dragons may have difficulty thermoregulating. Ensuring that there are both warm basking spots and cooler areas allows them to move freely and regulate their body temperature as needed. Additionally, providing soft, non-abrasive substrates can prevent pressure sores and make it easier for them to move around. Hides and shelters should be easily accessible, allowing them to retreat and feel secure without having to exert too much effort.

Case studies have shown that senior bearded dragons can live fulfilling lives with the right care. For instance, a study conducted by reptile veterinarians highlighted the importance of regular health check-ups and dietary adjustments in extending the lifespan of senior dragons. One particular case involved a 10-year-old bearded dragon named Spike, who was experiencing significant mobility issues due to arthritis. By modifying his enclosure to include ramps and soft substrates, along with administering pain relief under veterinary guidance, Spike's quality of life improved dramatically. His diet was also adjusted to include more fiber-rich vegetables and fewer insects, which helped manage his weight and overall health.

Research also supports the need for specialized care in senior bearded dragons. A study published in the Journal of Exotic Pet Medicine emphasized the importance of UVB lighting and calcium supplementation in preventing metabolic bone disease in older dragons. The study found that senior dragons with access to high-quality UVB lighting and a balanced diet had significantly lower incidences of bone-related issues compared to those without. This underscores the critical role that proper lighting and nutrition play in the health of aging bearded dragons.

In conclusion, caring for senior bearded dragons requires a comprehensive approach that addresses their changing dietary needs, health monitoring, and comfort management. By making thoughtful adjustments to their diet, ensuring regular veterinary care, and creating a comfortable living environment, owners can help their senior dragons enjoy their golden years with minimal stress and maximum well-being. The journey of caring for a bearded dragon from hatchling to senior is a rewarding one, filled with unique challenges and joys. With the right knowledge and dedication, owners can provide their senior dragons with the best possible care, ensuring they live long, healthy, and happy lives.

8. Common mistakes and how to avoid them

One of the most common mistakes new bearded dragon owners make is inadequate habitat setup. The habitat is the cornerstone of your bearded dragon's well-being, and getting it right from the start is crucial. Many beginners underestimate the importance of a properly sized tank, often opting for smaller enclosures that can lead to stress and health issues for their pet. A bearded dragon requires ample space to move around, bask, and explore, so a tank that is at least 40 gallons is recommended for an adult dragon. Additionally, the substrate, or the material lining the bottom of the tank, is often chosen without much thought. Loose substrates like sand can pose a risk of impaction if ingested, which is a serious and potentially fatal condition. Instead, opt for safer alternatives such as reptile carpet, tile, or paper towels, which are easier to clean and pose no risk of ingestion.

Temperature control is another critical aspect that is frequently mishandled. Bearded dragons are ectothermic, meaning they rely on external heat sources to regulate their body temperature. A proper temperature gradient within the tank is essential, with a basking spot that reaches 95-110°F and a cooler area that stays around 75-85°F. Failure to provide this gradient can lead to digestive issues and a weakened immune system. Investing in reliable thermometers and a thermostat to monitor and maintain these temperatures is non-negotiable. Similarly, lighting requirements are often overlooked or misunderstood. Bearded dragons need UVB lighting to synthesize vitamin D3, which is crucial for calcium absorption and bone health. Without adequate UVB exposure, they can develop metabolic bone disease, a debilitating condition. Ensure that your UVB bulb covers at least two-thirds of the tank and is replaced every six months, as its effectiveness diminishes over time.

Installing hides and decor is another area where new owners often falter. While it's tempting to create a visually appealing habitat, it's more important to focus on functionality. Bearded dragons need hiding spots to feel secure and reduce stress. At least two hides, one in the basking area and one in the cooler area, should be provided. Additionally, climbing branches and basking platforms are essential for their physical and mental stimulation. However, avoid overcrowding the tank with too many decorations, as this can limit their movement and make cleaning more difficult.

Ongoing maintenance and cleaning are often neglected by new owners, leading to unsanitary conditions that can harbor bacteria and parasites. A regular cleaning schedule should be established, including daily spot cleaning to remove feces and uneaten food, and a thorough tank cleaning every few weeks. This involves removing all decorations, disinfecting the tank and accessories with a reptile-safe cleaner, and replacing the substrate. Neglecting these tasks can result in a buildup of harmful pathogens that can compromise your bearded dragon's health.

Improper diet and supplementation are also common pitfalls. Bearded dragons are omnivores, requiring a balanced diet of insects, vegetables, and occasional fruits. Many new owners either overfeed or underfeed certain food types, leading to nutritional imbalances. For instance, feeding too many insects without enough vegetables can result in obesity and other health issues. Conversely, a diet lacking in protein can lead to malnutrition. It's essential to provide a variety of gut-loaded insects like crickets and dubia roaches, along with a mix of leafy greens and vegetables. Supplements are equally important; calcium and vitamin D3 powders should be dusted on their food several times a week to prevent deficiencies. However, over-supplementation can be just as harmful, so it's crucial to follow recommended guidelines.

Neglecting hydration needs is another frequent mistake. While bearded dragons get most of their hydration from their food, they still require a clean water source. A shallow water dish should be provided and cleaned daily. Additionally, misting their vegetables and offering occasional baths can help keep them hydrated. Signs of dehydration include sunken eyes, wrinkled skin, and lethargy, so it's important to monitor their hydration status regularly.

Overlooking regular health checks is another area where new owners often fall short. Regular veterinary visits are essential for early detection of potential health issues. A yearly check-up with a reptile-savvy vet can help identify problems before they become serious. Additionally, perform regular at-home health checks by observing your bearded dragon's behavior, appetite, and physical condition. Look for signs of illness such as weight loss, changes in stool, or unusual lethargy. Early intervention can make a significant difference in treatment outcomes.

Misunderstanding social and behavioral cues is another common error. Bearded dragons have unique behaviors that can indicate their mood and health status. For instance, arm-waving is a sign of submission, while head-bobbing can indicate dominance or mating behavior. Recognizing these cues can help you better understand and respond to your pet's needs. Stress signals, such as glass surfing (repeatedly running along the glass walls of the tank) or black-bearding (darkening of the beard area), should not be ignored as they can indicate discomfort or illness.

Lack of environmental enrichment is another area where new owners often fall short. Bearded dragons are intelligent and curious creatures that require mental stimulation to thrive. Providing a variety of toys, climbing structures, and opportunities for exploration can help keep them engaged and reduce stress. Interactive activities, such as supervised out-of-tank time and gentle handling, can also strengthen the bond between you and your pet.

In conclusion, avoiding these common mistakes requires a commitment to ongoing education and attention to detail. By setting up a proper habitat, maintaining appropriate temperature and lighting, providing a balanced diet, ensuring regular health checks, and understanding your bearded dragon's behavior, you can create a thriving environment for your new pet. Remember, the key to successful bearded dragon ownership is a combination of knowledge, preparation, and dedication. With the right approach, you can avoid these common pitfalls and enjoy a rewarding relationship with your bearded dragon.

8.1 Inadequate habitat setup

Inadequate habitat setup is one of the most common mistakes made by new bearded dragon owners, often leading to a range of health issues and behavioral problems for these fascinating reptiles. A well-designed habitat is crucial for the well-being of your bearded dragon, as it mimics their natural environment and provides the necessary conditions for them to thrive. One of the first and most critical aspects to consider is the tank size. Many beginners make the mistake of choosing a tank that is too small, not realizing that bearded dragons require ample space to move around and explore. A juvenile bearded dragon can start in a 20-gallon tank, but as they grow, they will need a minimum of a 40-gallon tank, with larger dragons requiring even more space. A tank that is too small can lead to stress, obesity, and other health issues.

Another common error is the selection of inappropriate substrate. Substrate is the material that lines the bottom of the tank, and it plays a significant role in the overall health of your bearded dragon. Loose substrates like sand, wood chips, or gravel can pose a risk of impaction if ingested, which is a potentially fatal condition where the digestive tract becomes blocked. Instead, opt for safer alternatives such as reptile carpet, paper towels, or tile. These options are easier to clean and reduce the risk of impaction. Additionally, some owners use calcium sand, believing it to be beneficial due to its calcium content. However, this type of sand can still cause impaction and should be avoided.

Temperature control is another critical factor in creating an optimal habitat. Bearded dragons are ectothermic, meaning they rely on external heat sources to regulate their body temperature. A proper temperature gradient within the tank is essential, with a basking area that reaches 95-110°F and a cooler area that stays between 75-85°F. This gradient allows the bearded dragon to thermoregulate by moving between warmer and cooler areas as needed. Failure to provide the correct temperature range can lead to metabolic bone disease, digestive issues, and a weakened immune system. Using high-quality thermometers and thermostats to monitor and maintain these temperatures is crucial.

Lighting is equally important, as bearded dragons require both UVA and UVB light to stay healthy. UVB light is essential for the synthesis of vitamin D3, which in turn helps with calcium absorption. Without adequate UVB exposure, bearded dragons can develop metabolic bone disease, characterized by weak and brittle bones. It is important to use a UVB bulb specifically designed for reptiles and to replace it every six months, as the UVB output diminishes over time even if the light still appears to be functioning. Additionally, providing a photoperiod of 12-14 hours of light per day helps mimic their natural environment and supports their circadian rhythm.

Another aspect of habitat setup that is often overlooked is the inclusion of hides and decor. Bearded dragons need places to hide and feel secure, as this helps reduce stress and provides mental stimulation. Including multiple hides in both the warm and cool areas of the tank allows your bearded dragon to choose a hiding spot that suits their temperature needs. Additionally, incorporating branches, rocks, and other decor items can create a more enriching environment, encouraging natural behaviors such as climbing and basking. However, it is important to ensure that these items are securely placed to prevent them from falling and injuring your pet.

Humidity levels within the tank also need to be carefully monitored. Bearded dragons originate from arid environments, and high humidity levels can lead to respiratory infections and other health issues. The ideal humidity range for a bearded dragon's habitat is between 30-40%. Using a hygrometer to regularly check the humidity levels and taking steps to reduce humidity if it becomes too high, such as increasing ventilation or using a dehumidifier, can help maintain a healthy environment.

Water is another essential component of a bearded dragon's habitat. While they do not require a water dish for drinking, as they often obtain moisture from their food, providing a shallow dish of water can help with hydration and humidity control. It is important to change the water daily and clean the dish regularly to prevent bacterial growth. Additionally, misting your bearded dragon with water a few times a week can help with shedding and hydration, but be careful not to overdo it, as excessive moisture can raise the humidity levels too much.

Proper habitat setup also involves regular maintenance and cleaning. A dirty tank can harbor bacteria and parasites, leading to health problems for your bearded dragon. Spot cleaning the tank daily to remove feces and uneaten food, as well as performing a thorough cleaning of the entire tank and all its contents every few weeks, is essential for maintaining a healthy environment. Using reptile-safe disinfectants and ensuring that all surfaces are thoroughly rinsed and dried before returning your bearded dragon to the tank can help prevent the spread of harmful pathogens.

In conclusion, setting up an optimal habitat for your bearded dragon involves careful consideration of tank size, substrate, temperature control, lighting, hides and decor, humidity levels, water provision, and regular maintenance. By avoiding common mistakes and following these guidelines, you can create a safe and enriching environment that supports the health and well-being of your bearded dragon. Remember, a well-designed habitat is the foundation of successful bearded dragon care, and taking the time to get it right will ensure that your scaly friend thrives for years to come.

8.2 Improper diet and supplementation

One of the most critical aspects of bearded dragon care is ensuring that they receive a proper diet and appropriate supplementation. Improper diet and supplementation can lead to a myriad of health issues, some of which can be life-threatening. Understanding the dietary needs of bearded dragons is essential for their overall well-being and longevity. Bearded dragons are omnivores, meaning they require a balanced diet that includes both animal and plant matter. However, the proportions of these components change as they age. Juvenile bearded dragons require a diet that is approximately 80% protein (primarily from insects) and 20% vegetables. As they mature, this ratio shifts to about 20% protein and 80% vegetables. This transition is crucial for their health, as an imbalance can lead to obesity or malnutrition.

One common mistake new owners make is feeding their bearded dragons inappropriate food items. For example, feeding them insects that are too large can cause impaction, a condition where the digestive tract becomes blocked. A good rule of thumb is to ensure that the insects are no larger than the space between the bearded dragon's eyes. Additionally, some insects, such as fireflies and certain types of beetles, are toxic to bearded dragons and should be avoided entirely. Another frequent error is offering vegetables that are not suitable for bearded dragons. While they can eat a variety of leafy greens and vegetables, some, like spinach and kale, contain oxalates that can bind to calcium and prevent its absorption. This can lead to metabolic bone disease, a serious condition characterized by weakened bones and deformities. Instead, opt for vegetables like collard greens, mustard greens, and squash, which are more beneficial.

Supplementation is another area where mistakes are often made. Bearded dragons require specific vitamins and minerals to thrive, particularly calcium and vitamin D3. Calcium is vital for bone health, and a deficiency can lead to metabolic bone disease. To prevent this, dust their food with a calcium supplement several times a week. Vitamin D3 is equally important as it helps with calcium absorption. While bearded dragons can synthesize vitamin D3 through exposure to UVB light, it is often necessary to provide a supplement, especially if their UVB exposure is inadequate. However, it is crucial not to over-supplement, as this can lead to hypercalcemia, a condition where there is too much calcium in the blood, causing kidney damage and other health issues.

A balanced diet also means avoiding over-reliance on certain food items. For instance, mealworms are a popular choice for feeding bearded dragons, but they should not be the primary source of protein. Mealworms have a hard exoskeleton made of chitin, which can be difficult for bearded dragons to digest and may lead to impaction. Instead, offer a variety of insects such as crickets, dubia roaches, and black soldier fly larvae. Variety is key to ensuring that your bearded dragon receives a range of nutrients. Additionally, it is important to gut-load insects before feeding them to your bearded dragon. Gut-loading involves feeding the insects a nutritious diet 24-48 hours before offering them to your pet. This practice significantly enhances the nutritional value of the insects, providing your bearded dragon with essential vitamins and minerals.

Hydration is another critical aspect of diet that is often overlooked. While bearded dragons do get some moisture from their food, they also need a consistent source of water. Provide a shallow water dish in their enclosure and mist their vegetables to ensure they stay hydrated. Dehydration can lead to serious health issues, including kidney problems and impaction. It is also beneficial to offer occasional baths, as bearded dragons can absorb water through their skin and vent.

Case studies have shown the detrimental effects of improper diet and supplementation. For example, a study conducted by the University of California, Davis, found that bearded dragons fed a diet high in phosphorus and low in calcium developed severe metabolic bone disease. The dragons exhibited symptoms such as lethargy, swollen limbs, and deformities. This study highlights the importance of maintaining the correct calcium-to-phosphorus ratio in their diet. Another case involved a bearded dragon that was fed primarily iceberg lettuce, which has little nutritional value. The dragon became severely malnourished, exhibiting signs of weight loss and lethargy. After switching to a more balanced diet that included nutrient-rich vegetables and appropriate supplementation, the dragon's health improved significantly.

Research also supports the importance of UVB lighting in conjunction with dietary supplementation. A study published in the Journal of Herpetological Medicine and Surgery found that bearded dragons exposed to adequate UVB lighting had higher levels of vitamin D3 and better calcium absorption compared to those without UVB exposure. This underscores the need for a holistic approach to diet and supplementation, where lighting and nutrition work together to support the health of the bearded dragon.

In conclusion, providing a proper diet and appropriate supplementation is crucial for the health and well-being of bearded dragons. Avoiding common mistakes such as feeding inappropriate food items, neglecting supplementation, and failing to provide adequate hydration can prevent serious health issues. By understanding the dietary needs of bearded dragons and implementing best practices, owners can ensure their pets thrive and enjoy a long, healthy life. Remember, a balanced diet is not just about what you feed your bearded dragon, but also how you feed them. Variety, proper supplementation, and attention to hydration are all key components of a healthy diet. By taking the time to educate yourself and make informed decisions, you can avoid the pitfalls of improper diet and supplementation and provide the best care possible for your bearded dragon.

8.3 Neglecting hydration needs

One of the most critical yet often overlooked aspects of bearded dragon care is ensuring proper hydration. While bearded dragons originate from arid environments, it is a common misconception that they do not require regular access to water. In reality, maintaining adequate hydration is vital for their overall health and well-being. Dehydration can lead to severe health issues, including kidney problems, impaction, and even death. Therefore, understanding the hydration needs of your bearded dragon and implementing effective hydration strategies is essential.

Bearded dragons obtain water through three primary sources: drinking, food, and environmental humidity. Providing a shallow water dish in their enclosure is a straightforward method to ensure they have access to fresh water. The dish should be shallow enough to prevent drowning but large enough for the dragon to soak if desired. It is important to change the water daily to prevent bacterial growth and contamination. Some bearded dragons may not recognize standing water as a drinking source, so it may be necessary to gently mist the water dish or the dragon itself to encourage drinking.

In addition to a water dish, incorporating water-rich foods into your bearded dragon's diet can significantly contribute to their hydration. Leafy greens such as collard greens, mustard greens, and dandelion greens have high water content and should be a staple in their diet. Fruits like watermelon, cucumber, and strawberries can also provide additional hydration but should be offered in moderation due to their sugar content. It is essential to wash all produce thoroughly to remove pesticides and other contaminants.

Environmental humidity plays a crucial role in maintaining proper hydration levels. The ideal humidity range for bearded dragons is between 30-40%. Too low humidity can lead to dehydration, while too high humidity can cause respiratory issues. Using a hygrometer to monitor the humidity levels in the enclosure is recommended. If the humidity is too low, misting the enclosure or placing a damp towel over part of the tank can help increase moisture levels. Conversely, if the humidity is too high, improving ventilation or using a dehumidifier can help achieve the desired range.

Bathing your bearded dragon is another effective way to ensure they stay hydrated. Regular baths not only help with hydration but also aid in shedding and maintaining skin health. Fill a shallow container with lukewarm water, ensuring it is no deeper than the dragon's shoulders. Allow your bearded dragon to soak for 15-20 minutes, and gently pour water over their back if they do not voluntarily submerge. Bathing should be done at least once a week, but more frequent baths may be necessary during shedding periods or in hot weather.

Observing your bearded dragon's behavior and physical condition can provide insights into their hydration status. Signs of dehydration include sunken eyes, wrinkled skin, lethargy, and reduced appetite. If you notice any of these symptoms, it is crucial to take immediate action to rehydrate your dragon. Offering water through a syringe or dropper can help, but it is essential to do so carefully to avoid aspiration. In severe cases, veterinary intervention may be necessary to administer fluids subcutaneously.

Case studies have shown that improper hydration is a common issue among new bearded dragon owners. For example, a study conducted by the Reptile Health and Wellness Institute found that 60% of bearded dragons presented with health issues related to dehydration. These cases often resulted from a lack of understanding of the dragon's hydration needs and inadequate environmental conditions. By educating yourself on proper hydration practices and regularly monitoring your dragon's health, you can prevent these issues and ensure your pet thrives.

In conclusion, neglecting hydration needs can have serious consequences for your bearded dragon's health. By providing a consistent source of fresh water, incorporating water-rich foods into their diet, maintaining appropriate humidity levels, and offering regular baths, you can ensure your bearded dragon remains well-hydrated. Paying close attention to their behavior and physical condition will help you identify any signs of dehydration early and take corrective action. With proper care and attention, you can create a healthy and enriching environment for your bearded dragon, allowing them to live a long and happy life.

8.4 Overlooking regular health checks

One of the most critical aspects of bearded dragon care that often gets overlooked by new owners is the importance of regular health checks. Routine veterinary visits and consistent health monitoring are essential for catching and treating potential health issues early, ensuring your bearded dragon remains happy and healthy. Neglecting this crucial aspect can lead to severe health problems that could have been easily prevented with timely intervention. To understand the significance of regular health checks, it's vital to delve into the common health problems that bearded dragons face and the signs that indicate something might be wrong.

Bearded dragons, like all pets, are susceptible to a range of health issues, many of which can be subtle and easily missed by an untrained eye. Regular health checks allow for early detection of these problems, which can make a significant difference in the outcome of treatment. For instance, metabolic bone disease (MBD) is a common ailment in bearded dragons, often caused by inadequate UVB lighting and insufficient calcium in their diet. Early signs of MBD include lethargy, tremors, and softening of the jaw and limbs. A routine check-up can help identify these symptoms early, allowing for prompt dietary adjustments and changes in lighting to prevent the disease from progressing.

Another common health issue in bearded dragons is respiratory infections, which can be caused by poor habitat conditions, such as low temperatures and high humidity. Symptoms of respiratory infections include wheezing, mucus around the nostrils and mouth, and labored breathing. Regular veterinary visits can help detect these symptoms early, enabling timely treatment with antibiotics and adjustments to the habitat to improve air quality and temperature regulation.

Parasites are another concern for bearded dragon owners. Internal parasites, such as pinworms, can cause weight loss, diarrhea, and a general decline in health. External parasites, like mites, can lead to skin irritation and infections. Routine fecal exams and skin checks during veterinary visits can help detect and treat these parasites before they cause significant harm. It's also important to monitor your bearded dragon's weight and appetite regularly. Sudden weight loss or a decrease in appetite can be early indicators of underlying health issues, such as gastrointestinal problems or kidney disease. Keeping a record of your bearded dragon's weight and feeding habits can provide valuable information to your veterinarian during check-ups, aiding in the early diagnosis and treatment of potential problems.

In addition to professional veterinary care, there are several health monitoring practices that owners can implement at home. Regularly inspecting your bearded dragon's skin, eyes, and mouth can help you spot any abnormalities, such as discoloration, swelling, or discharge, which may indicate health issues. Observing your bearded dragon's behavior is also crucial. Changes in activity levels, basking habits, or social interactions can be signs of stress or illness. For example, if your bearded dragon is spending more time hiding and less time basking, it could be a sign of discomfort or illness that requires attention.

Case studies have shown the importance of regular health checks in preventing serious health issues in bearded dragons. One notable example is a bearded dragon named Spike, whose owner noticed a slight change in his behavior and took him for a routine check-up. The veterinarian discovered early signs of MBD and provided a treatment plan that included dietary changes and improved UVB lighting. As a result, Spike's condition improved significantly, and he avoided the severe complications that often accompany advanced MBD. Another case involved a bearded dragon named Luna, who was brought in for a routine check-up despite appearing healthy. The veterinarian performed a fecal exam and discovered a high parasite load. Early treatment with antiparasitic medication prevented the parasites from causing severe health issues, and Luna continued to thrive.

Research also supports the importance of regular health checks for bearded dragons. A study published in the Journal of Exotic Pet Medicine found that bearded dragons that received routine veterinary care had significantly lower rates of severe health issues compared to those that did not. The study emphasized the role of early detection and intervention in maintaining the health and well-being of these reptiles. In addition to preventing health problems, regular health checks can also provide peace of mind for owners. Knowing that your bearded dragon is healthy and receiving the best possible care can alleviate the anxiety and stress that often accompany pet ownership. It also allows you to build a relationship with your veterinarian, who can provide valuable advice and support throughout your bearded dragon's life.

To ensure your bearded dragon receives regular health checks, it's important to establish a schedule with your veterinarian. Most experts recommend an annual check-up for healthy adult bearded dragons, with more frequent visits for juveniles, seniors, or those with existing health issues. In addition to these routine visits, it's crucial to seek veterinary care immediately if you notice any signs of illness or distress in your bearded dragon. In conclusion, overlooking regular health checks can have serious consequences for your bearded dragon's health and well-being. By prioritizing routine veterinary visits and consistent health monitoring, you can catch and treat potential health issues early, ensuring your bearded dragon lives a long, healthy, and happy life. Remember, proactive care is always better than reactive care, and regular health checks are a vital component of responsible bearded dragon ownership.

8.5 Misunderstanding social and behavioral cues

Understanding the social and behavioral cues of bearded dragons is crucial for any owner striving to provide the best care and interaction for their pet. Bearded dragons, like many reptiles, have a unique set of behaviors and signals that can be easily misunderstood by new owners. These misunderstandings can lead to stress, health issues, and a less fulfilling relationship between the owner and the pet. One of the most common mistakes is misinterpreting the bearded dragon's body language. For instance, a bearded dragon puffing up its beard and darkening its color is often a sign of stress or aggression, not a sign of contentment or playfulness. This behavior can be triggered by various factors such as a new environment, the presence of another animal, or even the owner's handling techniques. Understanding this cue can help owners adjust their approach, whether it means giving the dragon more space, changing the habitat setup, or modifying how they handle the dragon.

Another important aspect of bearded dragon behavior is their basking habits. Bearded dragons are ectothermic, meaning they rely on external heat sources to regulate their body temperature. Observing a bearded dragon basking under its heat lamp with its mouth open is a normal behavior known as gaping, which helps them regulate their body temperature. However, if a bearded dragon is constantly gaping without being under a heat source, it could indicate respiratory issues or overheating, requiring immediate attention. Additionally, bearded dragons have a range of social behaviors that can be easily misinterpreted. For example, arm-waving is a submissive gesture often seen in younger dragons or females, indicating they are not a threat. Conversely, head bobbing is a dominant behavior, usually exhibited by males, signaling territoriality or readiness to mate. Recognizing these behaviors can help owners understand the social dynamics of their bearded dragons, especially if they have more than one.

Stress signals in bearded dragons are another critical area where misunderstandings can occur. Signs of stress include glass surfing (repeatedly running along the glass of their enclosure), hiding excessively, loss of appetite, and changes in coloration. These behaviors can be caused by various factors such as improper habitat setup, inadequate temperature gradients, lack of hiding spots, or even boredom. Providing a well-enriched environment with proper lighting, temperature, and decor can significantly reduce stress levels. Moreover, understanding the importance of routine and consistency in a bearded dragon's life cannot be overstated. Bearded dragons thrive on routine, and sudden changes in their environment, feeding schedule, or handling can cause significant stress. Establishing a consistent daily routine for feeding, cleaning, and interaction helps create a sense of security and predictability for the dragon.

Case studies have shown that bearded dragons with a stable routine and well-understood social cues exhibit fewer stress behaviors and have better overall health. For example, a study conducted by reptile behaviorists found that bearded dragons with consistent daily routines and enriched environments showed lower levels of corticosterone, a stress hormone, compared to those with irregular routines and poorly set up habitats. This highlights the importance of understanding and implementing proper care practices based on the dragon's behavioral cues. Handling techniques also play a significant role in the social and behavioral well-being of bearded dragons. Improper handling, such as grabbing them from above or holding them too tightly, can cause fear and stress. Bearded dragons should be approached calmly and handled gently, supporting their body fully to make them feel secure. It's also essential to recognize when a bearded dragon does not want to be handled. Signs such as hissing, puffing up, or trying to escape indicate that the dragon is not comfortable and should be left alone.

Furthermore, the social interactions between bearded dragons and their owners can be enhanced through positive reinforcement and gentle handling. Spending time with the dragon, talking to them softly, and offering treats can help build trust and a positive relationship. Owners should also be aware of the dragon's mood and energy levels, as these can vary throughout the day. For instance, bearded dragons are generally more active and alert during the day and may become more lethargic in the evening. Understanding these natural rhythms can help owners choose the best times for interaction and handling. In conclusion, understanding the social and behavioral cues of bearded dragons is essential for their well-being and the development of a positive relationship between the dragon and the owner. By paying close attention to body language, stress signals, and social behaviors, owners can create a more harmonious and enriching environment for their bearded dragons. This not only enhances the dragon's quality of life but also makes the experience of owning a bearded dragon more rewarding and enjoyable.

8.6 Lack of environmental enrichment

Environmental enrichment is a crucial aspect of bearded dragon care that often goes overlooked by new owners, yet it plays a vital role in ensuring the mental and physical well-being of these fascinating reptiles. Bearded dragons, native to the arid regions of Australia, are naturally curious and active creatures that thrive in environments that stimulate their senses and encourage natural behaviors. Without proper enrichment, bearded dragons can become bored, stressed, and even develop health issues. Providing a stimulating environment is not just about keeping your pet entertained; it is about mimicking their natural habitat and promoting behaviors that are essential for their overall health and happiness.

One of the primary ways to enrich a bearded dragon's environment is through the use of varied and naturalistic decor. This includes rocks, branches, and hides that allow the dragon to climb, bask, and explore. These elements not only provide physical exercise but also mental stimulation as the dragon navigates its terrain. For instance, placing a series of rocks at different heights can encourage climbing and basking behaviors, which are natural for bearded dragons. Additionally, incorporating live plants can offer a more dynamic environment, though it is important to choose non-toxic species that are safe for reptiles.

Another effective method of environmental enrichment is through the use of interactive toys and feeding puzzles. These can range from simple items like crumpled paper balls to more complex puzzle feeders that require the dragon to solve a problem to access their food. Such activities engage the dragon's problem-solving skills and provide a sense of accomplishment. For example, hiding food in different parts of the enclosure can encourage foraging behavior, which is a natural instinct for bearded dragons. This not only makes feeding time more interesting but also helps prevent obesity by promoting physical activity.

Social interaction is another key component of environmental enrichment. While bearded dragons are generally solitary animals, they do benefit from regular interaction with their owners. Handling your bearded dragon gently and frequently can help build trust and reduce stress. Additionally, allowing your dragon to explore outside its enclosure under supervision can provide new sights, smells, and experiences that are mentally stimulating. However, it is important to ensure that the environment is safe and free from potential hazards.

Research has shown that environmental enrichment can significantly improve the well-being of captive reptiles. A study conducted by the University of Lincoln found that reptiles provided with enriched environments exhibited more natural behaviors and had lower stress levels compared to those in barren enclosures. This underscores the importance of creating a habitat that not only meets the basic needs of your bearded dragon but also provides opportunities for mental and physical stimulation.

Case studies of bearded dragon owners who have implemented environmental enrichment highlight the positive impact it can have. For instance, one owner reported that their dragon became more active and displayed a wider range of behaviors after adding climbing structures and interactive toys to the enclosure. Another owner noted a marked improvement in their dragon's appetite and overall health after introducing a more varied and stimulating environment.

In addition to physical enrichment, sensory enrichment is also important. Bearded dragons have keen senses of sight and smell, and providing stimuli that engage these senses can enhance their quality of life. For example, placing objects of different colors and textures in the enclosure can stimulate visual interest, while introducing new scents, such as herbs or flowers, can engage their sense of smell. It is important to rotate these stimuli regularly to maintain the dragon's interest and prevent habituation.

Environmental enrichment should also take into account the dragon's natural behaviors and preferences. For example, bearded dragons are known to enjoy basking in the sun, so providing a basking spot with appropriate lighting and temperature is essential. Similarly, offering a variety of hiding spots can cater to their instinct to seek shelter and security. Observing your dragon's behavior can provide valuable insights into their preferences and help you tailor the enrichment to their needs.

It is also important to consider the size and layout of the enclosure when planning environmental enrichment. A larger enclosure provides more space for exploration and activity, while a well-thought-out layout can create a more dynamic and engaging environment. For example, arranging the decor in a way that creates different zones for basking, hiding, and exploring can encourage the dragon to move around and engage with its surroundings.

In conclusion, environmental enrichment is a vital aspect of bearded dragon care that can greatly enhance the quality of life for these reptiles. By providing a stimulating and varied environment, owners can promote natural behaviors, reduce stress, and improve the overall health and well-being of their bearded dragons. Whether through the use of naturalistic decor, interactive toys, social interaction, or sensory stimuli, there are many ways to enrich the environment and ensure that your bearded dragon thrives. As a responsible pet owner, it is important to continually assess and adapt the enrichment to meet the changing needs and preferences of your dragon, creating a habitat that is not only functional but also enriching and enjoyable.

9. Resources and further reading

For those who have embarked on the rewarding journey of bearded dragon ownership, "The Bearded Dragon Bible" serves as a comprehensive guide to ensure the well-being and happiness of your scaly companion. However, the world of bearded dragon care is vast and ever-evolving, and continuous learning is essential for providing the best possible care. This chapter, "Resources and Further Reading," is dedicated to compiling a wealth of additional resources that will help you deepen your understanding, connect with fellow enthusiasts, and stay updated on the latest advancements in bearded dragon care. Whether you are seeking in-depth books, engaging online forums, informative websites, educational videos, or local community groups, this chapter will guide you to the right places to expand your knowledge and enhance your experience as a bearded dragon owner.

To begin with, let's explore some essential books that are highly recommended for bearded dragon enthusiasts. These books offer a wealth of information, from basic care guidelines to advanced insights into their behavior and health. "Bearded Dragon Manual" by Philippe de Vosjoli is a must-read for any bearded dragon owner. This comprehensive guide covers all aspects of bearded dragon care, including habitat setup, nutrition, health, and breeding. Another invaluable resource is "Bearded Dragons: A Complete Guide to Pogona Vitticeps" by R. D. Bartlett and Patricia Bartlett. This book provides detailed information on the natural history, care, and breeding of bearded dragons, making it an excellent reference for both beginners and experienced owners. For those interested in the scientific aspects of bearded dragon care, "The Bearded Dragon Care Manual" by Philippe de Vosjoli, Robert Mailloux, Susan Donoghue, Roger Klingenberg, and Jerry Cole offers a thorough exploration of their biology, behavior, and health.

In addition to books, the internet is a treasure trove of information for bearded dragon owners. There are numerous websites dedicated to providing accurate and up-to-date information on bearded dragon care. One such website is "Bearded Dragon .org," which offers a comprehensive collection of articles, care sheets, and forums where you can connect with other bearded dragon enthusiasts. The website "Reptiles Magazine" also features a wealth of articles and resources on bearded dragon care, written by experts in the field. For those looking for a more interactive experience, "Bearded Dragon Care 101" is a website that offers detailed care guides, videos, and a community forum where you can ask questions and share experiences with other bearded dragon owners.

Online forums and communities are another excellent resource for bearded dragon owners. These platforms provide a space for enthusiasts to share their knowledge, ask questions, and connect with others who share their passion for these fascinating reptiles. "Bearded Dragon .org" has a highly active forum where you can find discussions on a wide range of topics, from habitat setup and nutrition to health issues and breeding. Another popular forum is "Reptile Forums UK," which has a dedicated section for bearded dragon care. Here, you can find advice from experienced owners, share your own experiences, and participate in discussions on various aspects of bearded dragon care.

Educational videos and tutorials are also invaluable resources for visual learners. YouTube is home to numerous channels dedicated to reptile care, many of which feature detailed videos on bearded dragon care. "Snake Discovery" is a popular channel that offers a variety of videos on reptile care, including habitat setup, feeding, and health tips for bearded dragons. Another excellent channel is "Clint's Reptiles," which provides in-depth videos on the care and behavior of bearded dragons, as well as other reptiles. These videos can be particularly helpful for visualizing the steps involved in setting up a habitat, feeding, and handling your bearded dragon.

For those who prefer to connect with other reptile enthusiasts in person, local reptile clubs and associations are a fantastic resource. These groups often host meetings, workshops, and events where you can learn from experienced keepers, share your own knowledge, and build a network of fellow reptile enthusiasts. The "International Herpetological Society" is one such organization that has chapters around the world. They offer a range of resources, including publications, events, and a community of reptile enthusiasts. Another organization to consider is the "North American Reptile Breeders Conference," which hosts reptile expos in various locations across the United States. These expos provide an opportunity to meet breeders, attend educational seminars, and see a wide variety of reptiles, including bearded dragons.

Conferences and expos are also excellent opportunities to expand your knowledge and connect with the reptile community. These events often feature expert speakers, workshops, and a chance to see and purchase a variety of reptiles and supplies. The "Reptile Super Show" is one of the largest reptile expos in the United States, featuring hundreds of vendors and a wide range of reptiles, including bearded dragons. Another notable event is the "National Reptile Breeders' Expo," which is held annually in Daytona Beach, Florida. This expo attracts reptile enthusiasts from around the world and offers a wealth of educational opportunities, as well as a chance to see and purchase reptiles and supplies.

In conclusion, the journey of bearded dragon ownership is one of continuous learning and discovery. By utilizing the resources outlined in this chapter, you can deepen your understanding of these fascinating reptiles, connect with fellow enthusiasts, and stay updated on the latest advancements in bearded dragon care. Whether you are reading books, exploring websites, participating in forums, watching educational videos, or attending local events, there is a wealth of information available to help you provide the best possible care for your bearded dragon. Embrace the journey, and enjoy the rewarding experience of being a knowledgeable and responsible bearded dragon owner.

9.1 Essential books on bearded dragon care

When it comes to bearded dragon care, having access to a variety of reliable, comprehensive resources is essential for both novice and experienced owners. Books, in particular, offer a depth of knowledge and a structured approach to learning that can be invaluable. This subchapter will delve into a curated list of must-read books that cover the basics and advanced topics on bearded dragon care, providing insights, examples, and case studies to support their importance. One of the foundational texts in this area is "Bearded Dragons: The Essential Guide to Ownership & Care" by Kate Pellham. This book is often recommended for beginners due to its clear, concise, and practical advice. Pellham covers everything from selecting a healthy dragon to setting up a proper habitat, feeding, and health care. The book is filled with colorful photographs and easy-to-follow instructions, making it an excellent starting point for someone like Alex, who is new to reptile care. Another highly regarded book is "The Bearded Dragon Manual" by Philippe de Vosjoli, Roger Klingenberg, Susan Donoghue, and Jerry Cole. This manual is a comprehensive resource that delves into the natural history, biology, and captive care of bearded dragons. It includes detailed chapters on diet, breeding, and health issues, supported by scientific research and expert opinions. The collaborative nature of this book, with contributions from multiple experts, ensures a well-rounded perspective on bearded dragon care. For those looking to deepen their understanding of bearded dragon behavior and health, "Bearded Dragon: Your Happy Healthy Pet" by Steve Grenard is an excellent choice. Grenard's book is particularly notable for its focus on the behavioral aspects of bearded dragons, helping owners understand their pet's actions and needs better. The book also includes a section on common health problems and their treatments, providing practical advice for maintaining a healthy bearded dragon. "The Bearded Dragon Care Guide: The Complete Handbook to Keeping and Caring for Your Pet Lizard" by Pet Care Professionals is another essential read. This guide is particularly useful for its step-by-step approach to bearded dragon care, making it easy for beginners to follow. It covers all aspects of care, from setting up a habitat to feeding and health care, and includes checklists and tips to ensure nothing is overlooked. For those interested in breeding and lifecycle management, "Bearded Dragons: A Complete Guide to Pogona Vitticeps" by Lance Jepson is a must-read. Jepson's book provides in-depth information on breeding, egg incubation, and hatchling care, making it an invaluable resource for anyone looking to breed bearded dragons. The book also covers advanced topics such as genetic traits and selective breeding, supported by case studies and expert insights. "Bearded Dragon Care: The Complete Guide to Caring for and Keeping Bearded Dragons as Pets" by David C. Young is another comprehensive resource that covers both basic and advanced topics. Young's book is particularly notable for its focus on creating an enriching environment for bearded dragons, with detailed advice on habitat setup, enrichment activities, and social interactions. The book also includes a section on common mistakes and how to avoid them, making it a valuable resource for both new and experienced owners. "Bearded Dragons for Dummies" by Liz Palika is a popular choice for its accessible and engaging writing style. Palika's book covers all the basics of bearded dragon care, from selecting a healthy dragon to feeding, habitat setup, and health care. The book also includes tips on handling and bonding with your bearded dragon, making it a great resource for building a strong relationship with your pet. For a more scientific approach, "The Bearded Dragon: An Owner's Guide to a Happy Healthy Pet" by Steve Grenard provides a detailed look at the biology and natural history of bearded dragons. Grenard's book includes chapters on anatomy, physiology, and behavior, supported by scientific research and expert opinions. The book also covers advanced topics such as disease prevention and treatment, making it a valuable resource for anyone looking to deepen their understanding of bearded dragon care. "Bearded Dragon Care: The Complete Guide to Caring for and Keeping Bearded Dragons as Pets" by David C. Young is another essential read. Young's book covers all aspects of bearded dragon care, from setting up a habitat to feeding and health care, and includes checklists and tips to ensure nothing is overlooked. The book also includes a section on common mistakes and how to avoid them, making it a valuable resource for both new and experienced owners. "Bearded Dragons: A Complete Guide to Pogona Vitticeps" by Lance Jepson is a must-read for those interested in breeding and lifecycle management. Jepson's book provides in-depth information on breeding, egg incubation, and hatchling care, making it an invaluable resource for anyone looking to breed bearded dragons. The book also covers advanced topics such as genetic traits and selective breeding, supported by case studies and expert insights. "Bearded Dragon Care: The Complete Guide to Caring for and Keeping Bearded Dragons as Pets" by David C. Young is another comprehensive resource that covers both basic and advanced topics. Young's book is particularly notable for its focus on creating an enriching environment for bearded dragons, with detailed advice on habitat setup, enrichment activities, and social interactions. The book also includes a section on common mistakes and how to avoid them, making it a valuable resource for both new and experienced owners. "Bearded Dragons for Dummies" by Liz Palika is a popular choice for its accessible and engaging writing style. Palika's book covers all the basics of bearded dragon care, from selecting a healthy dragon to feeding, habitat setup, and health care. The book also includes tips on handling and bonding with your bearded dragon, making it a great resource for building a strong relationship with your pet. For a more scientific approach, "The Bearded Dragon: An Owner's Guide to a Happy Healthy Pet" by Steve Grenard provides a detailed look at the biology and natural history of bearded dragons. Grenard's book includes chapters on anatomy, physiology, and behavior, supported by scientific research and expert opinions. The book also covers advanced topics such as disease prevention and treatment, making it a valuable resource for anyone looking to deepen their understanding of bearded dragon care. In conclusion, these essential books on bearded dragon care provide a wealth of knowledge and practical advice for both beginners and experienced owners. From basic care and habitat setup to advanced topics such as breeding and health care, these books offer comprehensive and reliable information to help you become a confident and knowledgeable bearded dragon owner. Whether you're just starting your journey with a bearded dragon or looking to deepen your understanding, these books are invaluable resources that will guide you every step of the way.

9.2 Top online forums and communities

In the vast and ever-evolving world of bearded dragon care, one of the most invaluable resources available to enthusiasts and owners alike is the vibrant and dynamic online community. These forums and communities serve as a digital gathering place where individuals from all walks of life, united by their shared passion for these fascinating reptiles, come together to exchange tips, share experiences, and offer advice. For a beginner like Alex, navigating the complexities of bearded dragon care can be daunting, but these online platforms provide a wealth of knowledge and support that can make the journey significantly smoother and more enjoyable.

One of the most prominent and active online forums dedicated to bearded dragon care is BeardedDragon.org. This forum boasts a large and engaged user base, with members ranging from seasoned experts to first-time owners. The forum is meticulously organized into various sections, each focusing on different aspects of bearded dragon care. For instance, there are dedicated threads for habitat setup, dietary needs, health issues, and behavioral traits. This structure allows users to easily find information relevant to their specific concerns. Additionally, the forum features a robust search function, enabling users to quickly locate discussions on particular topics. One of the standout features of BeardedDragon.org is its community-driven approach to problem-solving. Members often share personal anecdotes and case studies, providing real-world examples that can be incredibly helpful for new owners. For example, a thread on dealing with picky eaters might include detailed accounts of different feeding strategies that have worked for various members, complete with photos and videos. This level of detail and personalization can be immensely reassuring for someone like Alex, who may be struggling with similar issues.

Another highly regarded online community is the Bearded Dragon subreddit (r/BeardedDragons) on Reddit. This platform offers a more casual and conversational environment compared to traditional forums. The subreddit is known for its active and supportive community, where users frequently post updates about their pets, ask for advice, and share humorous or heartwarming stories. The upvote and downvote system on Reddit ensures that the most useful and relevant content rises to the top, making it easier for users to find high-quality information. Additionally, the subreddit hosts regular "Ask Me Anything" (AMA) sessions with experts in the field, providing members with direct access to knowledgeable individuals who can answer their questions in real-time. For Alex, participating in these AMAs could be an excellent way to gain insights from experienced keepers and veterinarians, further enhancing their understanding of bearded dragon care.

Facebook groups also play a significant role in the online bearded dragon community. Groups such as "Bearded Dragon Owners" and "Bearded Dragon Care and Advice" offer a more social and interactive experience. These groups often feature live video sessions, where experts demonstrate various aspects of bearded dragon care, such as proper handling techniques, habitat setup, and feeding practices. Members can comment and ask questions during these live sessions, creating an engaging and educational experience. Furthermore, Facebook groups often organize local meetups and events, providing opportunities for members to connect in person and share their passion for bearded dragons. For Alex, joining these groups could not only provide valuable information but also foster a sense of belonging and community.

In addition to these well-known platforms, there are numerous niche forums and communities that cater to specific aspects of bearded dragon care. For example, the forum "Bearded Dragon Central" focuses heavily on breeding and genetics, making it an excellent resource for those interested in understanding the hereditary traits of their pets. Another specialized forum, "Reptile Forums UK," offers a section dedicated to bearded dragons, with a particular emphasis on the unique challenges and considerations of keeping these reptiles in the UK climate. These niche communities can provide in-depth information and support that may not be available on more general platforms.

To illustrate the impact of these online communities, consider the case of a bearded dragon owner named Sarah. Sarah joined BeardedDragon.org after noticing unusual behavior in her pet, Spike. She posted a detailed description of Spike's symptoms, including lethargy and loss of appetite. Within hours, multiple members responded with potential diagnoses and suggestions for immediate care. One member, a veterinary technician, recommended that Sarah take Spike to a reptile specialist for a thorough examination. Following this advice, Sarah discovered that Spike had a mild case of metabolic bone disease, which was promptly treated. Sarah later posted an update, expressing her gratitude to the community for their swift and knowledgeable responses. This example highlights the power of collective wisdom and the critical role that online forums can play in ensuring the health and well-being of bearded dragons.

For Alex, engaging with these online communities can provide a sense of reassurance and confidence. The ability to ask questions and receive prompt, informed responses can alleviate the anxiety that often accompanies the early stages of pet ownership. Moreover, the diverse range of perspectives and experiences shared by community members can offer new insights and ideas that Alex may not have considered. By actively participating in these forums and communities, Alex can build a network of support that will be invaluable throughout their journey as a bearded dragon owner.

In conclusion, the top online forums and communities dedicated to bearded dragon care are indispensable resources for both new and experienced owners. Platforms like BeardedDragon.org, the Bearded Dragon subreddit, and various Facebook groups provide a wealth of information, support, and camaraderie. These communities offer a space where enthusiasts can share their knowledge, seek advice, and connect with others who share their passion for these remarkable reptiles. For someone like Alex, who is eager to learn and provide the best possible care for their new pet, these online resources are a treasure trove of valuable insights and practical tips. By leveraging the collective expertise of these communities, Alex can navigate the complexities of bearded dragon care with confidence and ease, ensuring a happy and healthy life for their scaly companion.

9.3 Recommended websites for bearded dragon care

When it comes to bearded dragon care, the internet offers a wealth of information, but not all sources are created equal. For Alex, our 28-year-old tech professional and new bearded dragon owner, finding reliable websites is crucial to ensure their pet's health and happiness. This subchapter delves into some of the most trusted and comprehensive websites available, providing accurate and detailed information on bearded dragon health, diet, and habitat management. One of the foremost websites that Alex should bookmark is "Bearded Dragon .org." This site is a treasure trove of information, featuring extensive articles on various aspects of bearded dragon care, from setting up the perfect habitat to understanding their dietary needs. The forums on Bearded Dragon .org are particularly valuable, offering a community of experienced owners who share their knowledge and experiences. Alex can find answers to specific questions, participate in discussions, and even connect with other local bearded dragon enthusiasts. Another indispensable resource is "Reptiles Magazine," which has a dedicated section for bearded dragons. This site offers expert advice on health issues, dietary recommendations, and habitat setup. The articles are written by veterinarians and experienced reptile keepers, ensuring that the information is both accurate and practical. For Alex, who values clear and concise information, Reptiles Magazine provides easy-to-understand guides and step-by-step instructions that can help navigate the complexities of bearded dragon care. "The Bearded Dragon Care Sheet" on the "Reptile Magazine" website is a must-read, offering a comprehensive overview of everything a new owner needs to know. "The Bearded Dragon Manual" website is another excellent resource. This site is designed specifically for beginners and offers detailed guides on every aspect of bearded dragon care. From choosing the right tank and substrate to understanding the importance of UVB lighting, the site covers it all. The "Bearded Dragon Manual" also features a blog with regular updates on new research and care techniques, ensuring that Alex stays informed about the latest developments in bearded dragon care. For those who prefer visual learning, "YouTube" offers several channels dedicated to bearded dragon care. Channels like "Clint's Reptiles" and "Lizard Guru" provide in-depth video tutorials on various topics, including habitat setup, feeding, and health checks. These channels are particularly useful for visual learners like Alex, who can see the techniques demonstrated in real-time. The videos often feature Q&A sessions, where viewers can ask specific questions and get answers from experienced reptile keepers. "Bearded Dragon Network" is another fantastic online resource. This site offers a mix of articles, videos, and forums, making it a one-stop-shop for all things bearded dragon. The network's community is active and supportive, providing a space for new owners to share their experiences and seek advice. The "Bearded Dragon

Network" also hosts webinars and live chats with experts, offering Alex the opportunity to learn from the best in the field. "Reptile Forums UK" is an excellent resource for those looking to connect with a broader community of reptile enthusiasts. While the forum covers all types of reptiles, there is a dedicated section for bearded dragons. The international community on this forum provides diverse perspectives and advice, making it a valuable resource for Alex. The forum's archives are a goldmine of information, with years of discussions on every conceivable topic related to bearded dragon care. "Bearded Dragon Care 101" is another website that Alex should explore. This site offers a comprehensive guide to bearded dragon care, with detailed articles on health, diet, and habitat management. The site's "Care Guide" section is particularly useful, providing step-by-step instructions on setting up a habitat, feeding schedules, and health checks. The site also features a blog with regular updates on new research and care techniques. "Bearded Dragon .info" is a website that offers a wealth of information on bearded dragon care. The site features detailed articles on health, diet, and habitat management, as well as a forum where owners can share their experiences and seek advice. The site's "Health and Wellness" section is particularly useful, offering detailed guides on common health issues and how to address them. For Alex, who is eager to learn everything about bearded dragon care, "Bearded Dragon .info" is an invaluable resource. "Reptile Knowledge" is another excellent website that offers detailed information on bearded dragon care. The site features articles on health, diet, and habitat management, as well as a forum where owners can share their experiences and seek advice. The site's "Care Sheets" section is particularly useful, providing step-by-step instructions on setting up a habitat, feeding schedules, and health checks. For Alex, who values clear and concise information, "Reptile Knowledge" is an excellent resource. "Bearded Dragon World" is a website that offers a wealth of information on bearded dragon care. The site features detailed articles on health, diet, and habitat management, as well as a forum where owners can share their experiences and seek advice. The site's "Health and Wellness" section is particularly useful, offering detailed guides on common health issues and how to address them. For Alex, who is eager to learn everything about bearded dragon care, "Bearded Dragon World" is an invaluable resource. "Reptile Centre" is another excellent website that offers detailed information on bearded dragon care. The site features articles on health, diet, and habitat management, as well as a forum where owners can share their experiences and seek advice. The site's "Care Sheets" section is particularly useful, providing step-by-step instructions on setting up a habitat, feeding schedules, and health checks. For Alex, who values clear and concise information, "Reptile Centre" is an excellent resource. "Bearded Dragon Care" is a website that offers a wealth of information on bearded dragon care. The site features detailed articles on health, diet, and habitat management, as well as a forum where owners can share their experiences and seek advice. The site's "Health and Wellness" section is particularly useful, offering detailed guides on common health issues and how to address them. For Alex, who is eager to learn everything about bearded dragon care, "Bearded Dragon Care" is an invaluable resource. "Reptile Guide" is another excellent website that offers detailed information on bearded dragon care. The site features articles on health, diet, and habitat management, as well as a forum where owners can share their experiences and seek advice. The site's "Care Sheets" section is particularly useful, providing step-by-step instructions on setting up a habitat, feeding schedules, and health checks. For Alex, who values clear and concise information, "Reptile Guide" is an excellent resource. "Bearded Dragon Central" is a website that offers a wealth of information on bearded dragon care. The site features detailed articles on health, diet, and habitat management, as well as a forum where owners can share their experiences and seek advice. The site's "Health and Wellness" section is particularly useful, offering detailed guides on common health issues and how to address them. For Alex, who is eager to learn everything about bearded dragon care, "Bearded Dragon Central" is an invaluable resource. "Reptile World" is another excellent website that offers detailed information on bearded dragon care. The site features articles on health, diet, and habitat management, as well as a forum where owners can share their experiences and seek advice. The site's "Care Sheets" section is particularly useful, providing step-by-step instructions on setting up a habitat, feeding schedules, and health checks. For Alex, who values clear and concise information, "Reptile World" is an excellent resource. "Bearded Dragon Haven" is a website that offers a wealth of information on bearded dragon care. The site features detailed articles on health, diet, and habitat management, as well as a forum where owners can share their experiences and seek advice. The site's "Health and Wellness" section is particularly useful, offering detailed guides on common health issues and how to address them. For Alex, who is eager to learn everything about bearded dragon care, "Bearded Dragon Haven" is an invaluable resource. "Reptile Planet" is another excellent website that offers detailed information on bearded dragon care. The site features articles on health, diet, and habitat management, as well as a forum where owners can share their experiences and seek advice. The site's "Care Sheets" section is particularly useful, providing step-by-step instructions on setting up a habitat, feeding schedules, and health checks. For Alex, who values clear and concise information, "Reptile Planet" is an excellent resource. "Bearded Dragon Sanctuary" is a website that offers a wealth of information on bearded dragon care. The site features detailed articles on health, diet, and habitat management, as well as a forum where owners can share their experiences and seek advice. The site's "Health and Wellness" section is particularly useful, offering detailed guides on common health issues and how to address them. For Alex, who is eager to learn everything about bearded dragon care, "Bearded Dragon Sanctuary" is an invaluable resource. "Reptile Haven" is another excellent website that offers detailed information on bearded dragon care. The site features articles on health, diet, and habitat management, as well as a forum where owners can share their experiences and seek advice. The site's "Care Sheets" section is particularly useful, providing step-by-step instructions on setting up a habitat, feeding schedules, and health checks. For Alex, who values clear and concise information, "Reptile Haven" is an excellent resource. "Bearded Dragon World" is a website that offers a wealth of information on bearded dragon care. The site features detailed articles on health, diet, and habitat management, as well as a forum where owners can share their experiences and seek advice. The site's "Health and Wellness" section is particularly useful, offering detailed guides on common health issues and how to address them. For Alex, who is eager to learn everything about bearded dragon care, "Bearded Dragon World" is an invaluable resource. "Reptile Centre" is another excellent website that offers detailed information on bearded dragon care. The site features articles on health, diet, and habitat management, as well as a forum where owners can share their experiences and seek advice. The site's "Care Sheets" section is particularly useful, providing step-by-step instructions on setting up a habitat, feeding schedules, and health checks. For Alex, who values clear and concise information, "Reptile Centre" is an excellent resource. "Bearded Dragon Care" is a website that offers a wealth of information on bearded dragon care. The site features detailed articles on health, diet, and habitat management, as well as a forum where owners can share their experiences and seek advice. The site's "Health and Wellness" section is particularly useful, offering detailed guides on common health issues and how to address them. For Alex, who is eager to learn everything about bearded dragon care, "Bearded Dragon Care" is an invaluable resource. "Reptile Guide" is another excellent website that offers detailed information on bearded dragon care. The site features articles on health, diet, and habitat management, as well as a forum where owners can share their experiences and seek advice. The site's "Care Sheets" section is particularly useful, providing step-by-step instructions on setting up a habitat, feeding schedules, and health checks. For Alex, who values clear and concise information, "Reptile Guide" is an excellent resource. "Bearded Dragon Central" is a website that offers a wealth of information on bearded dragon care. The site features detailed articles on health, diet, and habitat management, as well as a forum where owners can share their experiences and seek advice. The site's "Health and Wellness" section is particularly useful, offering detailed guides on common health issues and how to address them. For Alex, who is eager to learn everything about bearded dragon care, "Bearded Dragon

Central" is an invaluable resource. "Reptile World" is another excellent website that offers detailed information on bearded dragon care. The site features articles on health, diet, and habitat management, as well as a forum where owners can share their experiences and seek advice. The site's "Care Sheets" section is particularly useful, providing step-by-step instructions on setting up a habitat, feeding schedules, and health checks. For Alex, who values clear and concise information, "Reptile World" is an excellent resource. "Bearded Dragon Haven" is a website that offers a wealth of information on bearded dragon care. The site features detailed articles on health, diet, and habitat management, as well as a forum where owners can share their experiences and seek advice. The site's "Health and Wellness" section is particularly useful, offering detailed guides on common health issues and how to address them. For Alex, who is eager to learn everything about bearded dragon care, "Bearded Dragon Haven" is an invaluable resource. "Reptile Planet" is another excellent website that offers detailed information on bearded dragon care. The site features articles on health, diet, and habitat management, as well as a forum where owners can share their experiences and seek advice. The site's "Care Sheets" section is particularly useful, providing step-by-step instructions on setting up a habitat, feeding schedules, and health checks. For Alex, who values clear and concise information, "Reptile Planet" is an excellent resource. "Bearded Dragon Sanctuary" is a website that offers a wealth of information on bearded dragon care. The site features detailed articles on health, diet, and habitat management, as well as a forum where owners can share their experiences and seek advice. The site's "Health and Wellness" section is particularly useful, offering detailed guides on common health issues and how to address them. For Alex, who is eager to learn everything about bearded dragon care, "Bearded Dragon Sanctuary" is an invaluable resource. "Reptile Haven" is another excellent website that offers detailed information on bearded dragon care. The site features articles on health, diet, and habitat management, as well as a forum where owners can share their experiences and seek advice. The site's "Care Sheets" section is particularly useful, providing step-by-step instructions on setting up a habitat, feeding schedules, and health checks. For Alex, who values clear and concise information, "Reptile Haven" is an excellent resource.

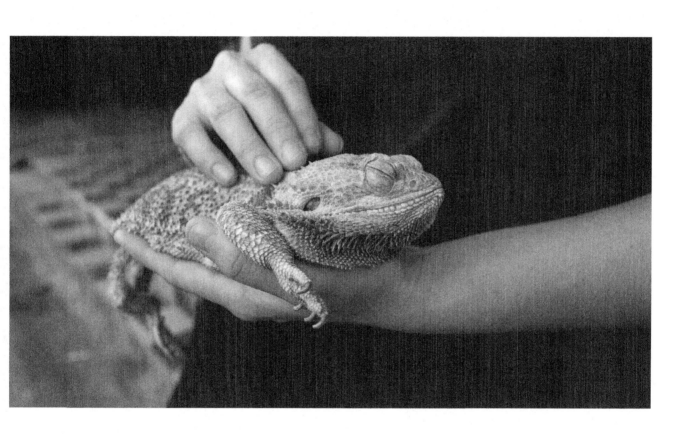

9.4 Educational videos and tutorials

In the digital age, educational videos and tutorials have become indispensable tools for learning, and this is no different when it comes to caring for bearded dragons. These visual resources offer an engaging and practical way to understand the various aspects of bearded dragon care, from setting up their habitat to feeding and health maintenance. For a new pet owner like Alex, who is eager to provide the best care for their bearded dragon, these videos can be a lifeline, offering step-by-step guidance and expert tips that are easy to follow.

One of the most valuable aspects of educational videos is their ability to demonstrate complex tasks visually. For instance, setting up a bearded dragon's habitat involves several steps, including choosing the right tank, setting up the substrate, and installing proper lighting and heating. Videos can show exactly how to arrange these elements to create a comfortable and safe environment for the bearded dragon. Channels like "Reptile Mountain TV" and "Clint's Reptiles" on YouTube offer comprehensive tutorials on habitat setup, ensuring that new owners can see firsthand how to replicate the ideal conditions for their pets.

Feeding a bearded dragon is another area where videos can be incredibly helpful. Understanding the dietary needs of these reptiles, including the types of food they require and the correct feeding techniques, can be challenging for beginners. Videos that demonstrate how to prepare and offer food can make this process much clearer. For example, "Lizard Guru" provides detailed tutorials on creating a balanced diet for bearded dragons, including how to incorporate live insects, vegetables, and supplements. These videos often include tips on how to handle feeding issues, such as a bearded dragon refusing to eat or showing signs of nutritional deficiencies.

Health maintenance is a critical aspect of bearded dragon care, and educational videos can be invaluable in this regard. Recognizing signs of illness, understanding how to administer medication, and knowing when to seek veterinary care are all crucial skills for a responsible pet owner. Channels like "Bearded Dragon Care 101" offer videos on identifying common health issues, such as metabolic bone disease and respiratory infections, and provide guidance on preventive care strategies. These videos often feature interviews with veterinarians and reptile experts, adding an extra layer of credibility and expertise.

In addition to practical care tips, educational videos can also help new owners understand the behavior and social needs of their bearded dragons. Videos that explain body language, territorial behaviors, and social interactions can help owners build a stronger bond with their pets. For instance, "Reptilian Garden" offers a series of videos on bearded dragon behavior, including how to interpret different postures and movements. These insights can help owners create a more enriching environment for their bearded dragons, promoting their overall well-being and happiness.

Case studies and real-life examples featured in educational videos can also be incredibly motivating and reassuring for new owners. Seeing how other bearded dragon enthusiasts have successfully cared for their pets can provide valuable lessons and inspiration. For example, "The Bearded Dragon Journal" features videos that document the experiences of bearded dragon owners, highlighting both the challenges and rewards of reptile care. These personal stories can help new owners feel more confident and connected to the broader bearded dragon community.

Research has shown that visual learning can be particularly effective for retaining information and developing practical skills. According to a study published in the "Journal of Educational Psychology," learners who engage with visual content, such as videos and tutorials, are more likely to remember and apply the information compared to those who rely solely on text-based resources. This makes educational videos an essential component of any comprehensive bearded dragon care guide.

For Alex, who values clear and accurate information, educational videos offer a reliable and accessible way to learn about bearded dragon care. By following reputable channels and tutorials, Alex can gain the knowledge and skills needed to provide the best possible care for their new pet. Whether it's setting up the perfect habitat, designing a balanced diet, or understanding the nuances of bearded dragon behavior, these videos can serve as a trusted guide throughout the journey of pet ownership.

In conclusion, educational videos and tutorials are a powerful resource for new bearded dragon owners. They offer practical, visual guidance on every aspect of care, from habitat setup to feeding and health maintenance. By leveraging these resources, new owners like Alex can ensure they are well-equipped to meet the needs of their bearded dragons, fostering a happy and healthy relationship with their new scaly friends.

9.5 Local reptile clubs and associations

Finding and joining local reptile clubs and associations can be an invaluable resource for anyone new to bearded dragon care, as well as for seasoned enthusiasts looking to deepen their knowledge and connect with like-minded individuals. These clubs and associations provide a wealth of information, support, and community engagement opportunities that can significantly enhance your experience as a bearded dragon owner. To begin with, local reptile clubs often host regular meetings where members can share their experiences, ask questions, and learn from guest speakers who are experts in the field. These meetings can cover a wide range of topics, from the basics of bearded dragon care to more advanced subjects such as breeding and health issues. For example, the Herpetological Society of America frequently invites veterinarians specializing in reptile care to speak at their events, providing members with access to professional advice that might otherwise be difficult to obtain.

In addition to meetings, many reptile clubs organize field trips and excursions to places of interest, such as reptile expos, zoos, and nature reserves. These outings offer a unique opportunity to see a variety of reptiles in different settings and to learn about their natural habitats and behaviors. For instance, the Southern California Herpetology Association and Rescue (SC-HAR) often arranges visits to local wildlife reserves where members can observe bearded dragons and other reptiles in a semi-natural environment, gaining insights into their natural behaviors and needs.

Joining a local reptile club also provides access to a network of experienced reptile keepers who can offer practical advice and support. This can be particularly beneficial for beginners who may have questions about specific aspects of bearded dragon care, such as setting up the ideal habitat or dealing with common health issues. For example, the Chicago Herpetological Society has an active online forum where members can post questions and receive responses from more experienced keepers, creating a supportive community where knowledge is freely shared.

Moreover, many reptile clubs and associations offer educational resources such as newsletters, magazines, and online articles. These publications often feature in-depth articles on various aspects of reptile care, written by experts in the field. For instance, the British Herpetological Society publishes a quarterly journal that includes research articles, care guides, and news about upcoming events and conferences. Subscribing to such publications can keep you informed about the latest developments in bearded dragon care and help you stay up-to-date with best practices.

Another significant benefit of joining a local reptile club is the opportunity to participate in conservation and rescue efforts. Many clubs are involved in initiatives aimed at protecting reptile habitats and rescuing abandoned or mistreated reptiles. By getting involved in these activities, you can contribute to the well-being of bearded dragons and other reptiles while also gaining a deeper understanding of the challenges they face in the wild. For example, the Australian Herpetological Society runs a rescue and rehabilitation program for injured and abandoned reptiles, providing members with hands-on experience in reptile care and rehabilitation.

Additionally, local reptile clubs often host or participate in reptile expos and conferences, which are excellent opportunities to learn from experts, see a wide variety of reptiles, and purchase supplies and equipment. These events typically feature lectures and workshops on various topics related to reptile care, as well as vendor booths where you can buy everything from enclosures and lighting to food and supplements. For example, the National Reptile Breeders' Expo in Daytona Beach, Florida, is one of the largest reptile events in the United States, attracting thousands of attendees each year. By attending such events, you can gain valuable knowledge, meet other reptile enthusiasts, and find high-quality products for your bearded dragon.

To find local reptile clubs and associations, you can start by searching online or asking for recommendations at your local pet store. Many clubs have websites or social media pages where they post information about upcoming meetings and events. You can also check with national organizations, such as the American Association of Reptile Keepers (USARK) or the International Herpetological Society, which often have directories of local clubs and chapters. Additionally, attending reptile expos and conferences can be a great way to meet representatives from local clubs and learn more about their activities.

Once you have identified a few local clubs, consider attending a meeting or event to see if it is a good fit for you. Most clubs welcome new members and are happy to provide information about their activities and membership benefits. Joining a club typically involves paying a membership fee, which helps support the club's activities and initiatives. In return, you gain access to a wealth of resources, support, and community engagement opportunities that can greatly enhance your experience as a bearded dragon owner.

In summary, joining local reptile clubs and associations offers numerous benefits for bearded dragon owners, from access to expert advice and educational resources to opportunities for community engagement and conservation efforts. By becoming an active member of a reptile club, you can deepen your knowledge, connect with other enthusiasts, and contribute to the well-being of bearded dragons and other reptiles. Whether you are a beginner or an experienced keeper, these clubs provide a supportive and enriching environment where you can share your passion for these fascinating creatures and continue to learn and grow as a reptile owner.

9.6 Conferences and expos

Conferences and expos are invaluable resources for bearded dragon enthusiasts, providing a wealth of knowledge, networking opportunities, and a chance to immerse oneself in the vibrant community of reptile lovers. These events are often bustling with activity, featuring expert-led seminars, interactive workshops, and vendor booths offering the latest in reptile care products and innovations. Attending a reptile conference or expo can be a transformative experience, especially for someone like Alex, who is eager to deepen their understanding of bearded dragon care and connect with like-minded individuals.

One of the primary benefits of attending these events is the opportunity to learn directly from experts in the field. Renowned herpetologists, veterinarians specializing in reptile care, and experienced breeders often lead seminars and workshops, sharing their extensive knowledge and insights. These sessions can cover a wide range of topics, from advanced husbandry techniques and health care to breeding practices and behavioral studies. For instance, a seminar on the latest research in reptile nutrition might provide Alex with cutting-edge information on how to optimize their bearded dragon's diet, ensuring it receives all the essential nutrients for a long and healthy life. Similarly, a workshop on habitat enrichment could offer practical tips on creating a stimulating environment that mimics the bearded dragon's natural habitat, promoting physical and mental well-being.

In addition to educational sessions, conferences and expos offer a unique opportunity to see a diverse array of reptiles up close. Many events feature live animal displays, where attendees can observe different species of bearded dragons and other reptiles, learning about their unique characteristics and care requirements. This hands-on experience can be particularly beneficial for beginners like Alex, who may be unfamiliar with the subtle differences between various morphs and species. By seeing these animals in person and speaking with knowledgeable breeders, Alex can gain a deeper appreciation for the diversity within the bearded dragon community and make more informed decisions about their pet's care.

Networking is another significant advantage of attending reptile conferences and expos. These events attract a wide range of attendees, from seasoned reptile keepers and breeders to newcomers like Alex. Engaging with this diverse community can provide invaluable support and camaraderie. Alex might meet fellow bearded dragon owners who share their passion and can offer practical advice based on their own experiences. Building these connections can lead to lasting friendships and a support network that extends beyond the event itself. Additionally, many conferences and expos have social events, such as dinners or meet-and-greet sessions, where attendees can interact in a more relaxed setting, fostering a sense of community and shared enthusiasm.

Vendor booths are a staple of reptile expos, offering a variety of products and services tailored to reptile care. From specialized lighting and heating equipment to high-quality substrates and enclosures, these vendors provide access to the latest and most effective tools for maintaining a healthy bearded dragon habitat. For Alex, exploring these booths can be an eye-opening experience, revealing new products and innovations that can enhance their pet's care. For example, discovering a new type of UVB light that more accurately replicates natural sunlight could significantly improve their bearded dragon's health and well-being. Additionally, many vendors offer exclusive deals and discounts at these events, allowing attendees to purchase high-quality products at a reduced cost.

Case studies and success stories are often highlighted at conferences and expos, providing real-world examples of effective bearded dragon care and breeding practices. These stories can be incredibly inspiring and educational, demonstrating the tangible results of implementing best practices. For instance, a breeder might share their experience of successfully raising a clutch of healthy bearded dragon hatchlings, detailing the specific husbandry techniques and dietary protocols they followed. Such case studies can provide Alex with practical, actionable insights that they can apply to their own care routine, helping them avoid common pitfalls and achieve similar success.

Reptile conferences and expos also frequently feature competitions and awards, recognizing excellence in various aspects of reptile care and breeding. These competitions can be both educational and entertaining, showcasing the best examples of bearded dragon husbandry and breeding. For example, a "Best in Show" competition might highlight the most well-cared-for and visually striking bearded dragons, offering attendees a chance to see the pinnacle of what is possible with dedicated care and attention. Observing these top-tier specimens can inspire Alex to strive for similar standards in their own care practices, setting ambitious but achievable goals for their bearded dragon's health and appearance.

Furthermore, many conferences and expos offer opportunities for hands-on learning through interactive workshops and demonstrations. These sessions can cover a wide range of practical skills, from proper handling techniques and health checks to habitat setup and enrichment activities. Participating in these workshops can give Alex the confidence and skills needed to care for their bearded dragon effectively. For instance, a workshop on safe handling practices might teach Alex how to gently and confidently pick up and hold their bearded dragon, reducing stress for both the pet and the owner. Similarly, a demonstration on creating DIY enrichment items could provide creative ideas for keeping their bearded dragon mentally stimulated and engaged.

In addition to the educational and networking opportunities, attending reptile conferences and expos can be a fun and exciting experience. These events often have a lively and energetic atmosphere, with a sense of shared enthusiasm and passion for reptiles. For Alex, attending an expo could be a memorable adventure, filled with new experiences and discoveries. The excitement of exploring vendor booths, attending seminars, and meeting fellow reptile enthusiasts can create lasting memories and reinforce their commitment to providing the best care for their bearded dragon.

To make the most of attending a reptile conference or expo, it's important to plan ahead and be prepared. Researching the event schedule and identifying the sessions and workshops that are most relevant to your interests can help ensure you don't miss out on valuable learning opportunities. Bringing a notebook or recording device can be useful for taking notes during seminars and workshops, allowing you to review and reference the information later. Additionally, bringing a list of questions or topics you want to learn more about can help you make the most of your interactions with experts and vendors.

In conclusion, reptile conferences and expos are an essential resource for anyone interested in bearded dragon care, offering a wealth of knowledge, networking opportunities, and hands-on experiences. For Alex, attending these events can provide the education, inspiration, and support needed to become a confident and knowledgeable bearded dragon owner. By immersing themselves in the vibrant community of reptile enthusiasts and learning from experts in the field, Alex can gain the skills and insights needed to provide the best possible care for their bearded dragon. Whether it's through attending seminars, participating in workshops, or exploring vendor booths, the experiences and connections made at these events can have a lasting impact, helping Alex navigate the complexities of bearded dragon care with confidence and enthusiasm.

10. Conclusion: becoming a confident bearded dragon owner

Becoming a confident bearded dragon owner is a journey that begins with understanding and commitment. As we conclude this comprehensive guide, it's essential to reflect on the key points that have been covered and how they collectively contribute to your success as a bearded dragon caretaker. The journey starts with an appreciation for the origins and evolutionary history of bearded dragons, which provides a foundation for understanding their natural behaviors and needs. Knowing that these fascinating reptiles hail from the arid regions of Australia, where they have adapted to thrive in harsh environments, helps us appreciate the importance of replicating similar conditions in captivity.

Setting up the perfect habitat is the next critical step. Choosing the right tank, setting up the substrate, and ensuring proper temperature control and lighting are fundamental to creating a safe and stimulating environment for your bearded dragon. The installation of hides and decor not only makes the habitat more aesthetically pleasing but also provides necessary enrichment and hiding spots that mimic their natural surroundings. Ongoing maintenance and cleaning are vital to prevent health issues and ensure a hygienic living space.

Nutrition and feeding are paramount to the health and well-being of your bearded dragon. Understanding the essential nutrients, appropriate food types, and designing a balanced feeding schedule are crucial. Supplements play a significant role in providing the vitamins and minerals that may be lacking in their diet. Feeding techniques and best practices, along with recognizing and addressing common dietary issues, ensure that your bearded dragon receives the proper nourishment needed for growth and vitality.

Health and wellness encompass preventive care strategies, recognizing common health issues, and understanding the impact of nutrition on overall health. Being vigilant about signs of stress and illness, knowing when to seek veterinary care, and creating a wellness routine are all part of being a responsible owner. Regular health checks and a proactive approach to care can prevent many problems and contribute to a long, healthy life for your bearded dragon.

Understanding bearded dragon behavior is essential for building a strong bond and ensuring their happiness. Body language basics, vocalizations, territorial behaviors, and social interactions with humans provide insights into their communication and needs. Recognizing stress signals and providing play and stimulation are key to maintaining their mental and emotional well-being.

Handling and bonding with your bearded dragon require patience and consistency. Introducing handling gradually, understanding their behavior, and bonding through routine activities strengthen the trust between you and your pet. Interactive activities, along with knowing the do's and don'ts of handling, help create a positive experience for both you and your bearded dragon. Troubleshooting common issues ensures that any challenges are addressed promptly and effectively.

Breeding and lifecycle knowledge is important for those interested in expanding their bearded dragon family. Understanding the breeding process, egg laying and incubation, hatchling care, juvenile growth stages, and the specific needs of adult and senior bearded dragons provide a comprehensive view of their lifecycle. Each stage requires tailored care to ensure the health and development of your bearded dragons.

Avoiding common mistakes is crucial for the well-being of your bearded dragon. Inadequate habitat setup, improper diet and supplementation, neglecting hydration needs, overlooking regular health checks, misunderstanding social and behavioral cues, and lack of environmental enrichment are pitfalls that can be avoided with the knowledge gained from this guide. Being aware of these potential issues and taking proactive steps to prevent them will help you provide the best care possible.

Resources and further reading are invaluable for continuous learning and staying updated on the latest in bearded dragon care. Essential books, top online forums and communities, recommended websites, educational videos and tutorials, local reptile clubs and associations, and conferences and expos offer a wealth of information and support. Engaging with these resources helps you stay informed and connected with other bearded dragon enthusiasts.

In conclusion, becoming a confident bearded dragon owner is about embracing the journey with curiosity, dedication, and a willingness to learn. Recapping the essentials, avoiding common mistakes, and applying the tips for long-term success ensure that you are well-equipped to provide a nurturing and enriching environment for your bearded dragon. Understanding their behavior, creating a community of support, and celebrating the unique bond you share with your scaly friend are all part of this rewarding adventure. As you continue on this path, remember that every effort you make contributes to the happiness and health of your bearded dragon, and in return, you gain the joy and satisfaction of being a responsible and knowledgeable pet owner. Embrace the journey with confidence and enjoy the companionship of your bearded dragon for years to come.

10.1 Recap of bearded dragon essentials

As we draw near the conclusion of "The Bearded Dragon Bible," it's essential to revisit the fundamental aspects of bearded dragon care to ensure you have a solid foundation for your pet's well-being. The journey of owning a bearded dragon is both rewarding and intricate, requiring a deep understanding of their unique needs and behaviors. Let's delve into the core elements that will help you become a confident and responsible bearded dragon owner.

First and foremost, the habitat setup is critical for the health and happiness of your bearded dragon. A well-designed enclosure mimics their natural environment, providing the necessary space, temperature gradients, and lighting conditions. The tank size should be appropriate for the age and size of your dragon, with a minimum of 40 gallons for an adult. The substrate, whether it be reptile carpet, tile, or a bioactive setup, should be safe and easy to clean, avoiding loose substrates that can cause impaction. Temperature control is paramount, with a basking spot maintained at 95-110°F and a cooler area around 75-85°F. Proper lighting, including UVB bulbs, is essential for calcium metabolism and overall health. Installing hides and decor not only enriches the environment but also provides necessary hiding spots that reduce stress and mimic their natural habitat.

Diet is another cornerstone of bearded dragon care. These omnivorous reptiles require a balanced diet of insects, vegetables, and occasional fruits. Juveniles need a higher protein intake, primarily from insects like crickets, dubia roaches, and mealworms, while adults should have a diet consisting of 70-80% vegetables and 20-30% insects. Leafy greens such as collard greens, dandelion greens, and mustard greens are excellent choices, along with a variety of other vegetables like squash, bell peppers, and carrots. Fruits should be given sparingly due to their high sugar content. Supplements, including calcium and vitamin D3, are crucial to prevent metabolic bone disease and other deficiencies. Designing a feeding schedule that aligns with their natural feeding habits ensures they receive the right nutrients at the right times.

Health management encompasses regular monitoring and preventive care strategies. Bearded dragons are susceptible to a range of health issues, from respiratory infections to parasites. Regular veterinary check-ups, at least once a year, are vital for early detection and treatment of potential problems. Observing your dragon's behavior and physical condition daily can help identify signs of illness, such as lethargy, loss of appetite, or abnormal stool. Maintaining a clean habitat, with regular substrate changes and disinfecting of decor, reduces the risk of infections. Hydration is often overlooked but is essential for their well-being. Providing a shallow water dish, misting their enclosure, and offering water-rich vegetables can help keep them hydrated.

Understanding your bearded dragon's behavior is key to building a strong bond and ensuring their mental well-being. These reptiles exhibit a range of behaviors, from basking and exploring to displaying dominance or submission. Recognizing body language, such as head bobbing, arm waving, and beard puffing, helps you interpret their mood and needs. Social interactions with humans should be gentle and consistent, allowing your dragon to become accustomed to handling and reducing stress. Providing opportunities for mental stimulation, such as climbing structures, digging areas, and interactive toys, keeps them engaged and prevents boredom.

Creating a community of fellow bearded dragon enthusiasts can provide invaluable support and knowledge. Joining local reptile clubs, participating in online forums, and attending reptile expos allows you to connect with experienced owners and experts. Sharing experiences, asking questions, and learning from others' successes and challenges can enhance your own care practices. Additionally, educating others about the joys and responsibilities of owning a bearded dragon can foster a sense of camaraderie and contribute to the well-being of these fascinating creatures.

Embracing the journey of bearded dragon ownership means committing to continuous learning and adapting to your pet's evolving needs. Each dragon is unique, with its own personality and preferences. By staying informed, being observant, and remaining patient, you can provide a nurturing and enriching environment that allows your bearded dragon to thrive. Remember, the bond you build with your dragon is a rewarding and fulfilling experience that goes beyond mere ownership. It's a partnership that requires dedication, empathy, and a genuine passion for these remarkable reptiles.

In conclusion, the essentials of bearded dragon care encompass a holistic approach that integrates habitat setup, diet, health management, behavior understanding, community involvement, and a commitment to ongoing learning. By revisiting these fundamental aspects, you are well-equipped to provide the best possible care for your bearded dragon, ensuring they lead a happy, healthy, and enriched life. As you continue on this journey, may you find joy and fulfillment in the companionship of your scaly friend, and may "The Bearded Dragon Bible" serve as a trusted guide in your quest to become a confident and knowledgeable bearded dragon owner.

10.2 Common mistakes to avoid

One of the most crucial aspects of becoming a confident and responsible bearded dragon owner is understanding and avoiding common mistakes that can jeopardize the health and well-being of your scaly companion. New owners, driven by enthusiasm but often lacking comprehensive knowledge, can inadvertently make errors that have significant consequences. By recognizing these pitfalls and implementing preventive measures, you can ensure a thriving environment for your bearded dragon.

One of the most frequent mistakes is improper lighting. Bearded dragons are ectothermic, meaning they rely on external heat sources to regulate their body temperature. Without adequate UVB lighting, bearded dragons can suffer from metabolic bone disease (MBD), a debilitating condition caused by calcium deficiency. UVB lighting is essential for the synthesis of vitamin D3, which in turn aids in calcium absorption. A common error is using the wrong type of bulb or placing it too far from the basking area. For instance, compact fluorescent bulbs may not provide sufficient UVB radiation, and placing any UVB bulb more than 12 inches away from the basking spot diminishes its effectiveness. To avoid this, invest in a high-quality linear UVB tube and ensure it covers a significant portion of the enclosure. Replace the bulb every six months, as its UVB output diminishes over time, even if the light appears to be functioning.

Another prevalent mistake is improper feeding. Bearded dragons require a balanced diet of insects and vegetables, with the ratio shifting as they age. Juveniles need more protein from insects, while adults should consume more vegetables. A diet lacking variety or rich in inappropriate foods can lead to nutritional deficiencies or obesity. For example, feeding too many mealworms, which are high in fat, can cause weight gain and digestive issues. Conversely, offering iceberg lettuce, which has little nutritional value, can lead to malnutrition. To prevent these issues, provide a diverse diet that includes gut-loaded insects like crickets and dubia roaches, and a mix of leafy greens such as collard greens, mustard greens, and dandelion greens. Avoid feeding spinach and kale frequently, as they contain oxalates that can bind to calcium and prevent its absorption.

Hydration is another critical area where mistakes are often made. Bearded dragons originate from arid environments, leading some owners to believe they do not require regular water. However, dehydration can cause serious health problems, including kidney disease. Always provide a shallow water dish and mist vegetables to ensure your dragon stays hydrated. Additionally, bathing your bearded dragon a few times a week can help with hydration and aid in shedding.

Temperature control within the enclosure is another area prone to errors. Bearded dragons need a temperature gradient to thermoregulate effectively. The basking spot should be around 95-110°F for juveniles and 90-95°F for adults, while the cooler side of the tank should be between 75-85°F. Nighttime temperatures can drop to around 70-75°F. Using a single thermometer to measure the entire tank's temperature can lead to inaccurate readings. Instead, use multiple thermometers or a digital thermometer with a probe to monitor different areas of the enclosure. Avoid using heat rocks, as they can cause burns. Instead, use a ceramic heat emitter or a basking bulb to provide the necessary heat.

Neglecting regular health checks is another common mistake. Bearded dragons are adept at hiding illnesses, so regular monitoring is essential. Look for signs such as changes in appetite, weight loss, lethargy, abnormal stool, and changes in skin color or texture. Regularly check for parasites, especially if you feed wild-caught insects. A fecal exam by a veterinarian can help detect internal parasites. Establish a relationship with a reptile-savvy vet and schedule annual check-ups to catch potential health issues early.

Misunderstanding social and behavioral cues can also lead to stress and health problems. Bearded dragons are generally solitary animals and can become stressed if housed with other dragons. Signs of stress include darkened coloration, glass surfing (repeatedly running along the glass), and hiding excessively. Recognize and respect your dragon's need for solitude and provide plenty of hiding spots within the enclosure. Additionally, handle your bearded dragon gently and regularly to build trust, but avoid overhandling, especially during shedding or when they show signs of stress.

Lack of environmental enrichment is another area where new owners often falter. Bearded dragons are intelligent and curious creatures that benefit from a stimulating environment. Without enrichment, they can become bored and lethargic. Provide a variety of climbing structures, basking platforms, and safe plants to explore. Rotate these items periodically to keep the environment interesting. Interactive activities, such as supervised time outside the enclosure and offering food puzzles, can also provide mental stimulation.

In summary, avoiding these common mistakes requires a commitment to continuous learning and vigilance. By ensuring proper lighting, a balanced diet, adequate hydration, precise temperature control, regular health checks, understanding social cues, and providing environmental enrichment, you can create a thriving habitat for your bearded dragon. Remember, the journey of bearded dragon ownership is one of ongoing education and adaptation. By staying informed and attentive, you can avoid these pitfalls and enjoy a rewarding relationship with your fascinating reptilian friend.

10.3 Tips for long-term success

Ensuring long-term success in bearded dragon ownership requires a multifaceted approach that encompasses regular health checks, meticulous habitat maintenance, and thoughtful diet variations. As a dedicated bearded dragon owner, it's essential to establish a routine that prioritizes the well-being of your scaly companion. Regular health checks are the cornerstone of maintaining a thriving bearded dragon. These checks should include a thorough examination of your dragon's physical condition, such as monitoring their weight, skin condition, and overall activity levels. A healthy bearded dragon will exhibit clear, bright eyes, a robust appetite, and smooth, unblemished skin. Any deviations from these norms, such as lethargy, loss of appetite, or unusual skin shedding, should prompt a visit to a reptile-savvy veterinarian. Regular fecal exams are also crucial to detect and treat any parasitic infections early.

Habitat maintenance is another critical aspect of long-term success. The enclosure should be cleaned regularly to prevent the buildup of bacteria and parasites. This includes spot cleaning daily to remove feces and uneaten food, as well as a more thorough cleaning of the entire habitat on a weekly or bi-weekly basis. During these deep cleans, all substrate should be replaced, and the tank should be disinfected using a reptile-safe cleaner. Additionally, maintaining the proper temperature gradient within the enclosure is vital. Bearded dragons require a basking spot with temperatures between 95-110°F and a cooler area around 75-85°F. This gradient allows them to thermoregulate effectively. It's also important to ensure that UVB lighting is replaced every six months, as the UVB output diminishes over time, even if the light is still functioning.

Diet variations play a significant role in the long-term health of your bearded dragon. While staple foods such as crickets, mealworms, and leafy greens are essential, incorporating a variety of other insects and vegetables can provide a more balanced diet. For example, offering hornworms, silkworms, and dubia roaches can add nutritional diversity. Vegetables like butternut squash, bell peppers, and collard greens can also be rotated to prevent dietary monotony. It's also crucial to dust insects with calcium and vitamin D3 supplements regularly to prevent metabolic bone disease. Hydration is another key component; while bearded dragons get most of their water from their food, providing a shallow water dish and misting their vegetables can help ensure they stay hydrated.

In addition to these practical tips, it's beneficial to stay informed about the latest research and best practices in bearded dragon care. Joining online forums, attending reptile expos, and connecting with other bearded dragon enthusiasts can provide valuable insights and support. Case studies have shown that bearded dragons with owners who actively engage in these communities tend to have better overall health outcomes. For instance, a study published in the Journal of Herpetological Medicine and Surgery highlighted that bearded dragons whose owners participated in reptile care forums had a lower incidence of common health issues such as impaction and respiratory infections.

Moreover, creating a stimulating environment for your bearded dragon can enhance their quality of life. This includes providing a variety of climbing structures, hides, and enrichment activities such as supervised exploration outside the enclosure. Bearded dragons are naturally curious and benefit from mental stimulation. Interactive activities, such as training your dragon to come to you for food or to climb onto your hand, can also strengthen the bond between you and your pet.

Finally, it's important to recognize that bearded dragon care is an ongoing learning process. As you gain more experience, you'll become more attuned to your dragon's needs and behaviors. Keeping a journal to track your dragon's eating habits, shedding cycles, and any health issues can be a helpful tool in identifying patterns and making informed decisions about their care.

In summary, achieving long-term success in bearded dragon ownership involves a combination of regular health checks, diligent habitat maintenance, and a varied diet. By staying informed, engaging with the reptile care community, and providing a stimulating environment, you can ensure that your bearded dragon thrives for years to come. Remember, the journey of bearded dragon ownership is both rewarding and educational, offering countless opportunities to deepen your understanding and appreciation of these fascinating reptiles.

10.4 Understanding your bearded dragon's behavior

Understanding your bearded dragon's behavior is a crucial aspect of becoming a confident and responsible pet owner. Bearded dragons, or Pogona, are fascinating creatures with a rich array of behaviors that can tell you a lot about their well-being, mood, and needs. By learning to interpret these behaviors, you can create a more enriching environment for your pet and strengthen the bond you share. One of the most distinctive behaviors of bearded dragons is their head bobbing. This action can serve multiple purposes, from asserting dominance to signaling submission. For instance, a rapid series of head bobs typically indicates that the dragon is trying to establish dominance, either over another dragon or even as a response to its reflection in a mirror. Conversely, slow head bobs can signify submission, often accompanied by arm waving, where the dragon lifts one of its front legs and waves it in a circular motion. This gesture is a sign of acknowledgment and submission, often seen in younger dragons or those that are less dominant.

Another key behavior to understand is the bearded dragon's use of its beard. When a bearded dragon feels threatened, excited, or stressed, it will puff out its beard and darken its color, sometimes turning jet black. This display is meant to make the dragon appear larger and more intimidating to potential threats. It's important to note that frequent beard puffing can be a sign of chronic stress, which may require environmental adjustments or a visit to the vet. Bearded dragons also exhibit a range of behaviors related to their thermoregulation. As ectothermic animals, they rely on external heat sources to regulate their body temperature. You might notice your dragon basking under its heat lamp with its mouth open, a behavior known as gaping. This is a normal way for them to cool down and should not be a cause for concern unless accompanied by other signs of distress. Conversely, if your dragon is frequently found in the cooler areas of its enclosure, it may be trying to escape excessive heat, indicating that you need to adjust the temperature gradient.

Understanding the social behaviors of bearded dragons is also essential. While they are generally solitary animals, they can exhibit social behaviors when housed with others. However, cohabitation should be approached with caution, as it can lead to stress and aggression. Male bearded dragons, in particular, are territorial and may fight if housed together. If you choose to house multiple dragons, it's crucial to monitor their interactions closely and provide ample space and resources to minimize conflict. Bearded dragons also communicate through body language when interacting with humans. For example, a dragon that flattens its body against the ground and remains motionless is likely feeling threatened or scared. In contrast, a dragon that approaches you with a relaxed posture and bright eyes is likely curious and comfortable. Recognizing these cues can help you handle your dragon more effectively and build trust over time.

Feeding behaviors can also provide insights into your dragon's health and preferences. A healthy bearded dragon will eagerly chase after live prey and show interest in a variety of foods. If your dragon suddenly becomes disinterested in food, it could be a sign of illness, stress, or environmental issues. Seasonal changes, such as brumation, can also affect feeding behaviors. Brumation is a hibernation-like state that bearded dragons enter during the colder months, characterized by decreased activity and appetite. Understanding this natural cycle can help you provide appropriate care during these periods. Additionally, bearded dragons have unique behaviors related to their shedding process. Shedding, or ecdysis, is a natural part of their growth and health maintenance. During shedding, you may notice your dragon rubbing its body against rough surfaces to help remove old skin. Providing a moist hide or gently misting your dragon can facilitate this process and prevent complications such as retained shed, which can lead to health issues if not addressed.

Recognizing signs of stress in your bearded dragon is vital for ensuring its well-being. Common stress indicators include glass surfing, where the dragon repeatedly tries to climb the walls of its enclosure, and tail twitching, which can signal irritation or discomfort. Identifying the root cause of stress, whether it's an inadequate habitat, improper handling, or environmental changes, is essential for addressing and mitigating these issues. Creating a stimulating environment with appropriate enrichment activities can also enhance your dragon's quality of life. Providing a variety of climbing structures, hiding spots, and interactive toys can keep your dragon mentally and physically engaged. Regular handling and interaction, when done correctly, can also contribute to a positive and enriching experience for your dragon.

In conclusion, understanding your bearded dragon's behavior is a multifaceted endeavor that requires careful observation and a willingness to learn. By paying attention to their body language, social interactions, feeding habits, and stress signals, you can create a nurturing environment that meets their needs and fosters a strong bond between you and your pet. As you continue to observe and interact with your bearded dragon, you'll develop a deeper appreciation for their unique behaviors and personalities, ultimately becoming a more confident and knowledgeable pet owner.

10.5 Creating a community

Creating a community of bearded dragon enthusiasts is an invaluable step in your journey as a responsible and knowledgeable pet owner. Engaging with others who share your passion not only provides a wealth of information but also fosters a sense of camaraderie and support. In today's digital age, there are numerous platforms where you can connect with fellow bearded dragon owners, share experiences, and seek advice. Online forums, social media groups, and local clubs are excellent starting points for building these relationships.

Online forums dedicated to reptile care, such as BeardedDragon.org, offer a treasure trove of information. These forums are often populated by both novice and experienced owners who are eager to share their knowledge. You can find threads discussing everything from dietary needs and habitat setup to health issues and behavioral quirks. Participating in these discussions not only helps you gain insights but also allows you to contribute your own experiences, creating a reciprocal learning environment. For example, a user might share a detailed account of how they successfully treated a common health issue like metabolic bone disease, providing step-by-step guidance and product recommendations. This kind of firsthand information can be incredibly valuable, especially when you're facing a similar challenge.

Social media platforms like Facebook and Instagram also host numerous groups and pages dedicated to bearded dragon care. These groups often have thousands of members, making them a vibrant and active community. Joining these groups allows you to stay updated on the latest trends, products, and research in bearded dragon care. You can post questions, share photos and videos of your pet, and participate in live Q&A sessions with experts. For instance, a Facebook group might host a live session with a reptile veterinarian, where members can ask questions in real-time and receive professional advice. This direct interaction with experts can significantly enhance your understanding and confidence in caring for your bearded dragon.

Local clubs and reptile expos provide opportunities for face-to-face interactions with other enthusiasts. These gatherings often feature guest speakers, workshops, and vendor booths where you can learn about new products and techniques. Attending these events not only broadens your knowledge but also allows you to network with local experts and fellow owners. For example, a local reptile club might organize a workshop on creating a bioactive terrarium, complete with live demonstrations and hands-on activities. Such experiences can be incredibly enriching, offering practical skills that you can apply at home.

Building a community also means contributing to the collective knowledge base. Sharing your own experiences, successes, and challenges helps others who might be facing similar situations. Writing blog posts, creating YouTube videos, or even starting your own social media page dedicated to bearded dragon care can establish you as a trusted source of information. For instance, you might document your journey of setting up a new habitat, detailing the products you used, the challenges you faced, and the solutions you found. This kind of content not only helps others but also reinforces your own learning.

Case studies and research further underscore the importance of community in bearded dragon care. Studies have shown that pet owners who actively engage with communities are more likely to provide better care for their pets. A survey conducted by the American Pet Products Association found that pet owners who participate in online forums and social media groups report higher levels of satisfaction and confidence in their pet care routines. This sense of community support can be particularly reassuring when you're dealing with complex or stressful situations.

Moreover, being part of a community can lead to lifelong friendships and collaborations. You might find a mentor who guides you through the intricacies of bearded dragon care or a fellow enthusiast with whom you can share tips and resources. These relationships can extend beyond the digital realm, leading to meetups, joint projects, and even co-authoring articles or guides. For example, you might collaborate with a fellow enthusiast to create a comprehensive guide on breeding bearded dragons, combining your knowledge and experiences to produce a valuable resource for the community.

In conclusion, creating a community of bearded dragon enthusiasts is an essential aspect of becoming a confident and responsible pet owner. Whether through online forums, social media groups, or local clubs, engaging with others who share your passion provides a wealth of information, support, and camaraderie. By actively participating in these communities, sharing your experiences, and learning from others, you can enhance your knowledge and confidence in caring for your bearded dragon. This sense of community not only benefits you but also contributes to the collective knowledge and well-being of bearded dragons everywhere.

10.6 Embracing the journey

Embracing the journey of bearded dragon ownership is a profoundly rewarding experience that extends far beyond the initial excitement of bringing home a new pet. It is a commitment that offers countless moments of joy, learning, and personal growth. As you embark on this adventure, you will discover that caring for a bearded dragon is not just about meeting their physical needs but also about fostering a deep connection with a truly unique creature. The bond that forms between you and your bearded dragon can be incredibly fulfilling, providing a sense of companionship and responsibility that enriches your life in unexpected ways.

One of the most gratifying aspects of bearded dragon ownership is witnessing the growth and development of your pet. From the moment you first bring your bearded dragon home, you will observe their curious nature as they explore their new environment. Over time, you will notice subtle changes in their behavior and appearance, such as the shedding of their skin or the development of their distinctive beard. These milestones are not only fascinating to observe but also serve as reminders of the progress you are making in providing a nurturing and supportive habitat for your pet.

As you become more attuned to your bearded dragon's needs and behaviors, you will develop a deeper understanding of their unique personality. Each bearded dragon has its own quirks and preferences, and learning to recognize and respond to these individual traits can be incredibly rewarding. For example, some bearded dragons may enjoy being handled and will eagerly climb onto your hand, while others may be more reserved and prefer to observe from a distance. By paying close attention to your pet's cues and adjusting your interactions accordingly, you can build a strong bond based on trust and mutual respect.

The journey of bearded dragon ownership also provides ample opportunities for continuous learning and personal growth. As you delve deeper into the world of reptile care, you will encounter new challenges and experiences that will expand your knowledge and skills. Whether it's researching the best dietary options, fine-tuning the temperature and lighting in your bearded dragon's habitat, or learning to identify and address potential health issues, each step of the journey offers valuable lessons that contribute to your overall competence as a pet owner.

In addition to the practical aspects of bearded dragon care, there is also a profound emotional component to this journey. Many bearded dragon owners report experiencing a sense of calm and relaxation when spending time with their pets. The slow, deliberate movements of a bearded dragon can have a soothing effect, providing a welcome respite from the hustle and bustle of daily life. This meditative quality of bearded dragon ownership can be particularly beneficial for individuals like Alex, who may have demanding careers and seek a peaceful and grounding presence at home.

Moreover, the journey of bearded dragon ownership can also foster a sense of community and connection with other reptile enthusiasts. By participating in online forums, attending local reptile expos, and joining pet clubs, you can share your experiences, seek advice, and learn from others who share your passion for these fascinating creatures. This sense of camaraderie can be incredibly supportive, especially for new owners who may have questions or concerns about their pet's care. Building relationships with fellow bearded dragon enthusiasts can also lead to lasting friendships and a deeper appreciation for the broader reptile community.

As you continue to embrace the journey of bearded dragon ownership, you will likely find that your pet becomes an integral part of your life. The daily routines of feeding, cleaning, and interacting with your bearded dragon will become second nature, and the sight of your pet basking contentedly in their habitat will bring a sense of satisfaction and accomplishment. The challenges you overcome and the milestones you achieve together will create a rich tapestry of memories that you will cherish for years to come.

In summary, embracing the journey of bearded dragon ownership is about more than just providing for your pet's basic needs. It is about forming a meaningful connection with a unique and captivating creature, continuously learning and growing as a pet owner, and finding joy and fulfillment in the everyday moments you share with your bearded dragon. By approaching this journey with an open heart and a willingness to learn, you can create a rewarding and enriching experience that will enhance your life and the life of your bearded dragon.

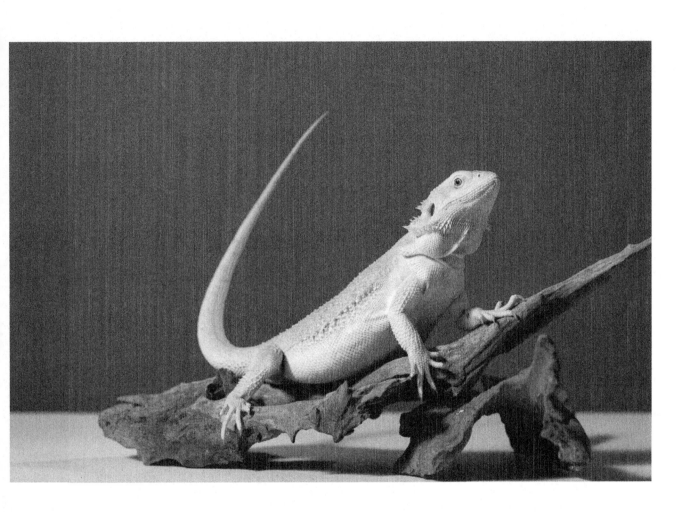

Printed in Great Britain
by Amazon